Praise for Kim Bensen and *Finally Thin!*

Donna Brinker, age 56, lost 115 lbs.

"Kim's book and website have been like finding an old, trusted friend. Her words have been encouraging, sincere, and filled with faith. I am a weight loss leader, also. But when I found myself struggling with my own weight issues again and starting to burn out, Kim's energy, passion, and faith made all the difference in helping me regain a positive 'can do' attitude! She is now my new 'old trusted friend.' Thanks, Kim!"

Holly Patkowski, age 37, lost 120 lbs.

"Kim has helped me on each step of my weight loss journey. She has motivated and inspired me to lose over 120 pounds, but she is also a huge encouragement while maintaining my weight loss as well. She is such a joy and light in my life, and I am so grateful that I found her book and her website!"

Pat Humeniuk, age 53, lost 48 lbs.

"Kim Bensen has taught me so much, not only about weight loss, but about life—mostly by her example. She welcomed me into her life through her book, *Finally Thin,* and then her weight-loss meetings and her online program. As if by magic that helped me turn my life around. A more kind and caring person will be hard to find."

Wendy Sebas, age 60, lost 62 lbs.

"From the moment I first met Kim, I trusted her completely. She taught me to believe in myself and to enjoy the journey. I am a slow loser and because of her never-ending encouragement, I am now 62 pounds lighter and finally at my weight goal! I would follow her anywhere. If you are looking for success, you've found it in Kim."

Luci Boyd, age 60, lost 33 lbs.

"I was sixty years old. I had no job, my knees hurt, and I was very overweight. Then I read *Finally Thin*. It gave me the motivation I needed to NOT give up. I lost 33 lbs and today, my knees no longer hurt and I feel great. Thank you, Kim!"

Phyllis McKinley, age 66, lost 34 lbs.

"I remember vividly the day I saw Kim on TV for the first time. I said aloud, 'She is going to be able to help me!' I eagerly awaited *Finally Thin,* her amazing book, arriving at my home. I have never read anything more honest, sincere, loving, or better researched. Kim was so open about her own challenges. Although I laughed and cried with her, my first thought was, *I can do this*—something I hadn't said for years! She has become a dear friend, and I am honored to be one of her beloved 'Kimmies.'"

finally thin!

finally

kim bensen

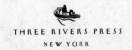

THREE RIVERS PRESS
NEW YORK

thin!

how i lost over

200 pounds

and kept them off—and how you can too

Copyright © 2008, 2010 by Kim Bensen

Published in the United States by Three Rivers Press, an imprint of the
Crown Publishing Group, a division of Random House, Inc., New York.
www.crownpublishing.com

THREE RIVERS PRESS and the Tugboat design are registered trademarks of
Random House, Inc.

Originally published in hardcover in slightly different form in the United States
by Broadway Books, an imprint of the Crown Publishing Group, a division of
Random House, Inc., New York, in 2008.

Library of Congress Cataloging-in-Publication Data

Bensen, Kim.
    Finally thin! : how I lost over 200 pounds and kept them off—and how you
can too / by Kim Bensen.—1st ed.
        p.   cm.
    (alk. paper)
    1. Weight loss.   I. Title.
    RM222.2.B4445   2009
    613.2'5—dc22   2008023730

ISBN 978-0-7679-2951-6
eISBN 978-0-7679-3150-2 (eBook)

PRINTED IN THE UNITED STATES OF AMERICA

Book design by Ralph Fowler / rlf design
Cover photographs: main photograph © Deborah Feingold; photo strip courtesy of the author

10 9 8 7 6 5 4 3 2 1

First Paperback Edition

for mark

From the . . .
moment I saw you on that stage in Colorado 34 years ago
time we met at Houghton 31 years ago
day were married 26 years ago
until today

Every time you . . .
say my name (what, 20 times since we were married?)
found money to pay a bill when there was none
showed tough love to the kids when I would have caved
paid for a new diet plan for me that would most likely end in weight gain
wink at me

You . . .
make me laugh :)
have handled financial hardship with honesty
fought heart disease, juvenile diabetes, and leukemia with courage
live your faith
made me feel beautiful at 350 pounds
amaze me

NNBILYM
1 Corinthians 13

contents

disclaimer

finally thin!

introduction

A friend once told me a joke about two elderly ladies sitting on a bench. One says to the other, "Did you hear that Helen died last week?" The other one sighs and says, "Yes, and only two pounds from her goal."

I chuckle every time I remember this story, but at the same time, don't you just wonder, "Will that be me? Will my weight-loss goal always elude me?"

Losing weight isn't the whole problem though, is it? We've all lost dozens, perhaps hundreds, of pounds in our lifetimes. The first problem is losing *all* of it, and the second problem is *keeping* it off. Over the years, that's something I had never been able to do, until now.

I finally did it and it's still hard to believe. After a lifetime of being overweight, I'm FINALLY THIN. Did I say I was thin? Wow! It's still a rush. I've only been *chubby, overweight,* or *morbidly obese* my entire life. I have to tell you there's nothing like hopping out of bed (yes, I did say *hopping*), slipping into jeans, and tucking in a T-shirt. Not wondering if it will fit. Not looking for a larger shirt that comes down over my butt. It's quick and easy and just feels so darn good that I really wanted to share that feeling with others.

For years *I* was the one glued to the television set every time another success story was about to come on. I grabbed the newest weight loss planners, tried all the fad diets, and rejoined Weight Watchers so many times I felt more like an investor than a member. So what was different this time? What did it take to stay motivated?

Before I go any further, I want you to understand something important: I am no different from you when it comes to losing weight. I don't have more willpower than you do. I don't lose weight more easily than you do. I'm a wife, a mom of four, and a businesswoman who faces the very same kinds of stresses and challenges that you do every day. I don't care how many times you've tried before, what drastic measures you've taken, and how downtrodden and discouraged you are right now. What matters is *not* your past; it's what lies ahead. Whether you're older or younger, richer or poorer, heavier or thinner than I was when I began, and whether you've tried to lose weight a bajillion times before to no avail, I truly believe *you can do this.*

Wouldn't it be fantastic to stop pulling in your stomach or hiding behind your children every time someone wanted to take your picture?

Wouldn't it be terrific to slide into *any* chair without worrying about whether you'll fit?

Wouldn't it be something if you could finally enjoy looking at your reflection in a store window or a full-length mirror?

I'm sure you've got your own list of frustrations, humiliations, and struggles that you'd like to put behind you. As you read my story in the following pages, you'll see that I had plenty of my own.

Finally Thin is *not* a weight-loss program. There are enough of those out there. Some really good ones as a matter of fact! *Finally Thin is* a book of motivation. And you can *never* have enough of that! It's a *concept* of how to find the program that best fits *you,* whether counting calories or carbs or Points or exchanges, and tailoring it to fit your lifestyle.

The fact is, all weight-loss programs are written for the masses. It's crucial to learn how to make yours enjoyable and satisfying for *you* and still get the results you desire, while discovering how to weave your chosen program throughout your daily life so that it becomes who you are and how you live. *That's* how to get all the way to your goal. *That's* how to keep the weight off forever. You end up living it and loving it so you want to keep on doing it. Not living on a diet—but learning how to tailor your diet to how you want to live. Only then can it become your lifestyle.

Today I'm a weight-loss leader giving weekly live meetings to thousands online at kimbensen.com. Some are following my calorie-counting program. Others are members at Weight Watchers; still others follow Atkins. But the way one person follows Weight Watchers is different from the way others do it. It HAS to be that way! We're all different people with different needs, taste buds, and schedules. There's no one diet, and no one way to "do" a diet that's right for everyone.

If you are reading this book, you are most likely one of the people who *have* to watch their weight. That stinks. Plain and simple. I know. Me, too. The fact is, if you choke down three small, tasteless meals in a 1,200-calorie day you will lose weight, but you probably won't want to eat that way for long and you'll give up *again,* eventually gaining the weight back. If, however, you eat delicious, satisfying meals that *you really like* in a 1,200-calorie day, you will lose weight, and you will be much more inclined to continue it long-term. The only thing is, no one knows exactly what appeals to *you* but *you.*

This book is broken down into three sections:

- First, my personal weight-loss story. It's a brutally honest recounting of my ups and downs (so to speak). The abandoned diets, the binges, the broken chairs, and the broken dreams. My all-consuming desire to be thin and healthy more than anything in the world, yet my continuing behavior of self-destruction over and over again. *But it's also a story of victory.* Of living a miraculous transformation, both inside and out, from a size 6X to a size 6. It's how I went from silently begging for help—to break free from the bondage of food—to finding myself in the position to be able to offer hope to others.

- The second section starts with a clear discussion of the basics of weight loss, so that whatever diet you follow, you'll know what is happening with your body. My Diet Shoppe then walks you through a straightforward description of all the major diets out there, with a thought-provoking quiz to help you choose which diets might best fit you. This brings you to *the 10 steps to a finally thin life*—ten steps to help weave your diet into the enjoyable, healthy lifestyle you've always wanted. It closes with tips and suggestions for making maintenance a reality.

- In the third section, you'll find dozens of my own delicious, family-tested recipes that don't taste like diet food—but will make your weight-loss journey a truly luscious one. I'm not a gourmet cook. In fact, my husband says, "Are you sure you don't want to call it the *I Can't Cookbook*?" (So much for spousal support.) But honestly, if it's too time-consuming, too difficult, or too hard to pronounce, most people won't make it. My recipes are all about yummy, every-day dishes that you can serve to the whole family and they won't even know they're eating light.

Finally thin . . . it *is* possible. Come on, it's YOUR turn now!

my story

the early years

I cringed as I heard my mother's quick steps heading down the rickety wooden stairs to the basement. I was in for it now. The basement was where we kept the spare freezer. The spare freezer was where mom kept boxes of Ring Dings, Twinkies, Funny Bones, and Sara Lee coffee cakes (as well as the extra staples). I knew what was coming next.

"Kimberly! May I see you please?" I could hear the frustration in her voice. For the past few weeks I had been carefully opening one side of each box and gingerly sliding out several packages before repositioning the boxes back with the open ends facing inward. I knew eventually she would run out of treats upstairs and head to the basement, discovering my theft. I was in junior high and couldn't seem to stop eating. Why did I keep doing it? What was the matter with me?

what's wrong with me, anyway?

Back then, I was the only person in my immediate family with a weight problem. Although members of my dad's extended family were obese, my dad was always thin. My mom was never heavy, and she made sure she stayed toned using the then-popular Royal Canadian Air Force Exercise Plan.

The plan was simply a slim paperback book, with a few photos and

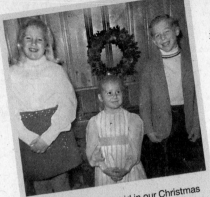

Me, Heather, and David in our Christmas photo in 1969. I always felt "big" next to my athletic brother and petite sister.

illustrations. Page after page described in detail what we kids thought were torturous exercises. Mom did these on the floor each morning for twenty minutes after Dad had gone to work. I vividly remember her "walking" across the bedroom floor on her buttocks, leaning back with her knees bent. *Right cheek. Left cheek.* None of us could keep up with her and, amusing as she was to watch, we rarely joined in. She never missed a day—and she never had a weight problem.

My brother, David, was just a year and two days older than me and was very athletic. MVP in football, soccer superstar. Baseball, basketball, you name it: David was good at it. He and my ballerina sister, Heather (four and a half years my junior), both had small frames and small appetites to go with them.

Not me.

While I was growing up, I was always focused on what was for dinner, how it was cooked, how much I got, and who got what was left over.

My earliest realization that food mattered more to me than to the other kids around me was at age eight. There I was, with six of my neighborhood pals, standing in our kitchen on Whittier Street in Andover, Massachusetts. My mom had just picked up some Chocolate Éclair ice cream bars, which she doled out to each of us. It was the first time I had ever tried this treat, and I immediately loved the light chocolaty crunch under its cake crumb exterior. When the other kids finished their ice cream, they thanked my mom and headed back outside to play.

Where were they going? *There were still more Éclairs in the box.* I knew! I had counted! I don't know what bothered me more—the fact that I desperately wanted another Éclair, or that all the other neighborhood kids had been satisfied with just one. I spent the next several minutes in a losing argument, begging my mother for another one before following my friends outdoors.

Shortly after that incident, I became aware of my actual weight as a number on the scale. I was sitting on a backyard jungle gym chatting with a girlfriend. I had just been to the doctor's office for a checkup and discovered that I weighed ninety-nine pounds. Even *I* knew that that was a lot for a nine-year-old. My friend told me that she weighed a lot less. I felt so embarrassed, and for the first time I didn't want anyone to know what my weight was.

By the time I entered fourth grade, my dad's job as a professional engineer had brought us to Ridgewood, New Jersey, where my mother signed me up for Weight Watchers. Although I was not obese, she knew that my extra weight bothered me. I was nine years old and into *Tiger Beat* magazine, Donny Osmond, and lip gloss. But my daydreams of Donny singing "Puppy Love" to me didn't mesh with the reality of my chubby physique.

When my mother had asked me if I'd like to give Weight Watchers a try, I jumped at the chance. *Get thin? Sure, I'll try anything!* Mom did all the figuring out and food preparation. All I had to do was eat the meals she made. The poor woman tried unsuccessfully to get me to eat liver once a week—then a Weight Watchers requirement. She went with me to all the weekly meetings. Even though I felt as if I were the only one there under seventy years old, I enjoyed going. One time, I was sitting in the meeting room with all the other women, who always had so much to share. The leader asked if anyone else had had a moment of triumph over food that week. I raised my hand and told in detail how I spit out a chewed-up chocolate bar in the sink rather than swallow it. I was so proud!

For years I would look back at the memory and cringe that I had actually shared that story. I probably grossed them all out, but they smiled and clapped anyway. Maybe it's age, or a new perspective, but today, as a Weight Watchers leader, I chuckle and think how proud I would be for any youngster to have such success. Still, my overall experience at Weight Watchers that first time was a positive one.

After a few months I'd lost about twelve pounds and stopped going to the meetings. I bought new clothes, and boys started paying more attention to me. I don't remember the weight coming back on, but it must have eventually, because by the time I got to junior high, I was again looking for ways to lose weight. My mom had just gotten a part-time job as a typesetter and, for the first time in my life, I was purchasing food at the cafeteria instead of brown-bagging it. That was when I discovered buttered hard rolls.

going up!

As a preteen, although I wasn't really fat, I also wasn't one of those willowy girls the boys went crazy for. My brother and I were best friends. We did everything together. I ate like the guys, played like the guys, and could throw a football like the guys—I was a true tomboy.

But I was beginning to wish I weren't one.

I joined the cheerleading squad. It was a perfect fit for me. I could be active and feminine and have a front-row seat at all my brother's football games. Without even trying, I got into great shape—until winter came and the activity stopped.

In high school I learned the real art of dieting. I lost and gained the same twenty pounds over and over again in a yo-yo cycle that would plague me for the next twenty-five years of my life. When I was a size 9 I felt wonderful; when I was a size 12 I felt awful. I did what all the girls did—skipped breakfast, pushed food around my plate at dinner. I even learned about making myself throw up from a girlfriend at summer camp. Fortunately, I wasn't very good at it and stopped before it became a long-term problem.

By the time I got to high school, my mother began "watching her weight" for the first time. We were living in Shelton, Connecticut, where Mom started her own typesetting business, working out of our home. Several of the women who worked for her also wanted to lose weight, and it seemed that they were trying a new fad diet every week. Each time someone decided to start something new, everyone else would jump on board—including me.

I tried all the hot diets featured in the tabloids: the apple-a-day diet, the grapefruit diet, diets where I fasted for two days in a row, and diets where I ate every three hours. Even though I was only fifteen to twenty pounds overweight, I talked my doctor into a prescription for diet pills, which worked great—until the prescription ran out.

It became a way of life, shifting from one diet to the next as I fasted and choked down some horrible concoctions. There were some really memorable ones. My girlfriend Sissy and I decided to begin a diet and walking program together. But before starting we decided to have one last binge. We headed for the grocery store and bought bags of our favorite cookies, cakes, and candy. By the time we were done eating, we were so sick we could barely move. That was the end of our "diet."

I'll say this for myself, I kept trying—and I tried *everything*.

Our family started attending Calvary Church in nearby Trumbull, where I found good friends and a strong faith in God. I learned a lot, read the Bible, and memorized some wonderful verses about overcoming temptation and asking God for help. But as much as I wanted to be free from the power that food seemed to have over me, I kept giving in.

Maybe exercise would be the key to losing the weight. Colorful exercise leotards, stretchy leg warmers, and matching sweatbands were all the rage in the late seventies as women began joining gyms in droves. My mom, her good friend and co-worker Shirl Jacobsen, and I joined a Gloria Stevens exercise salon, where aerobic classes and "pound pools" ruled our days. (A pound pool is a contest between dieters who each put some cash into the pot and then try to lose the most weight in order to win.) I knew how to lose quickly and won a lot of money taking off the same fifteen pounds over and over again.

losing weight, getting bigger

My life was defined by a pattern of gains and losses. This went on through my years in college, and eventually the spread of fifteen pounds grew to forty. On a few occasions, I found myself close to two hundred pounds. *Unthinkable!* But I was good at dieting and I was always able to get down to a somewhat comfortable weight again and again.

I lived the extremes, either consuming only celery sticks and salads or bingeing on Twinkies and fast food. There was no happy medium. I don't think my weight ever stayed the same for more than a week or two. It was either diet or binge, lose or gain, all or nothing, year after year after year.

I made the cheerleading squad again in college, though I joke that I was always at the bottom of the pyramid, never on the top. Being active helped, but the physical exercise I got was constantly offset by poor food choices.

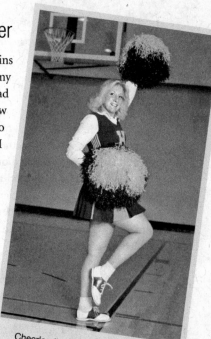

Cheerleading helped with my weight loss—at Houghton College in 1981. I was a cheerleader, but always at the bottom of the pyramid.

At Houghton College in upstate New York, I met my husband, Mark. At five feet, nine inches, and only 165 pounds, Mark was a trim, blond-haired, blue-eyed Norwegian with a great sense of humor and a kind, gentle personality.

We were both communications majors and had lots of classes to-

my story

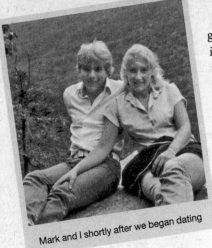
Mark and I shortly after we began dating

gether; many were group projects requiring hours of team research and study. He was my argument and debate partner and my speech "coach." Because we were both blonds, a few of our classmates commented on how much alike we looked.

"Don't you know that we're twins?" was Mark's quick comeback. He didn't even blink an eye. I went along with it, hiding a chuckle. No one even questioned him, so for two semesters everyone thought my last name was Bensen and that Mark was my twin brother.

He was so much fun to be with that I started sitting with him at meals and helping him at the radio station, where he was the program director. In a few months' time, Mark had become my best friend. I didn't want anything to change. I loved the closeness and ease of our relationship and didn't want romance to spoil that.

But my heart had other ideas. As much as I didn't want to, I was falling in love with my best friend and "twin brother." He had given me no indication that he wanted anything more than friendship, and I was content for a while to adore him secretly. But it was getting harder and harder. He got notes from friends at home—from girls. I felt a burning in my stomach that I had never felt before.

Mark was only a few inches taller than I was, so I started buying shoes that had a lower heel. I even lost weight, not wanting his thighs to be smaller than mine. I started wearing clothes with him in mind. *Would Mark like this? What would Mark think?*

It got to the point where I had to say something. Even though I feared ruining our wonderful friendship, I finally told him how I felt. It took me three hours one afternoon. After I blurted it all out, I couldn't believe it when he told me he felt the same way. He had just been waiting for me to realize that I was ready for more. Imagine the stir we caused on campus when the Bensen twins started dating!

love, marriage, and making a life with mark

Despite my newfound romance, my weight still fluctuated—from college cheerleader to binge eater and back again. One year I went to the spring banquet in a size 16 dress, the next year in a size 10. Through it all, though, Mark loved me.

After college, Mark went home to New Jersey and started working for a small broadcasting company. I joined my mom in her flourishing type-setting and graphic design business back in Shelton, Connecticut. Long-distance dating was hard on our pre–cell phone, pre-Internet relationship. As a result, Mark and I were engaged twice before we were married.

I bought my size 8 wedding dress during the first engagement. After a temporary pause in our romance, we got back together and were finally married on August 25, 1984. The second engagement was rather rushed to accommodate family plans. My sister was flying back to college at the end of the summer, so it was either rush a wedding or wait until Christmas vacation. We decided to rush, but that gave us only eight weeks to pull it off.

It was a crazy, busy time, but we had the "advantage" of having been engaged before, so many of the decisions had already been made. Everything else in life got put on hold, including my diet and exercise.

No one but Mom and I knew my dress had been let out three inches on each side just days before the wedding.

A week before the wedding, I tried on my gown. I couldn't believe it—it didn't fit! I was now a size 12—two sizes larger than the year before. I went to my mother in tears. Seven days later, I walked down the aisle with lace inserts pieced into the sides of my lovely gown. It looked fine and no one knew . . . except the bride and her mom.

life on a diet

After we got married, more than ever my life became a succession of diets, a pattern of losing and gaining weight over and over again. I tried almost everything—Weight Watchers (dozens of times), TOPS (Take Off Pounds Sensibly), OA (Overeaters Anonymous), Atkins, Slim-Fast, over-the-counter diet pills, prescription diet pills, Diet Center (loved their bran muffins!), the Weigh Down Workshop, hypnosis, even aversion therapy (complete with a staple in my ear—I don't recommend it).

When those didn't work, I purchased food plans and counted calories, bought weeks of packaged meals, and fasted for three months on a medically supervised fast. I worked out at Believersize (aerobics set to Christian music), Curves, and several other local gyms.

The amazing thing was, they all worked! Each one had a plan that, if adhered to, produced weight loss. But with each new diet I followed the same pattern: the excitement of beginning again, with a fresh start and a clean slate—perfection. *It almost seems easy. Why didn't I do this before? I can do this!* This brought a series of successful weigh-ins. Then, the inevitable breakdown. A bite of this, a taste of that. Not measuring, not keeping my food journal. And with that, the honeymoon was over. I did less and less planning and preparation, and the weight loss slowed to a halt. What had been so easy only a few weeks before had become torture to sustain.

My days would start out the same, each morning a new resolve. But they'd end up the same, too, with tears on my pillow, wondering why I had lost my willpower after starting out so strong.

If I could only "get it back."

I know I can do this.

I was doing it!

What's wrong with me?!

I'll be really good this week and lose enough to get back to where I was.

I would skip a meeting, not wanting my weigh-in book to show a gain. Thus, I would miss the very meeting I needed the most and continue on a downward spiral. In the end, I would never go back. And with each subsequent failure I just grew larger and more discouraged.

the down side of plus size

The more weight I gained, the harder life became. I had a range of clothing sizes in my wardrobe and was forever looking for something that fit me. I had to stop shopping in "normal" clothing stores and instead purchased all of my clothes at plus-size shops. I felt ashamed when I couldn't fit into a size 14 or 16 anymore. At the time, there just weren't many larger sizes in most department stores.

Fortunately for me, America was gaining weight as rapidly as I was. Before long, independent plus-size stores began opening in all the malls. Suddenly every department store had a "Women's" shop, and many major designers started making clothes for the larger woman. But even though it became easier to find clothes in my larger size, I lived in what I called my "uniform"—a pair of stretch pants (with stirrups in the early years) and a coordinating top that was long enough to cover my stomach and most of my buttocks. Whenever I found something that fit me and was flattering, the first question I asked was, "How many colors does this come in?"

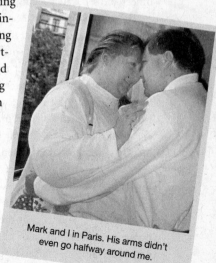

Mark and I in Paris. His arms didn't even go halfway around me.

Through it all, Mark never made a derogatory comment about my weight. He held me when I cried about how miserable I felt. He supported me whenever I began a new program and comforted me when I inevitably slipped off the wagon, but he also knew he couldn't lose the weight for me.

A year and a half after our marriage, our daughter, Aleeta, was born. Two years later, we had Adam. With each pregnancy, I was so sick with nausea for nine months that I couldn't hold anything down and actually lost weight each time. The only time in my life I didn't gain weight was when I was dieting or pregnant.

While I continued working with my mother in her graphics firm, Mark and I decided to start our own advertising agency and for twelve years we ran both businesses successfully out of a professional building in the downtown Shelton area. Aleeta and Adam practically grew up there. Most days after school, they would lie on the floor of the art department drawing, doing homework, and using up all our expensive art supplies to make superhero costumes. The three of us would head home for supper, often grabbing a delicious Shelton Pizza on the way. Mark would join us a little later.

Just when life seemed to have settled down, my dad's career required a move to Michigan. My parents sold the building. Mark and I merged the two businesses and moved the company into our home. Our house was built on a slightly sloping piece of property, which enabled us to build offices and separate parking in the lower walk-out level of our house.

About the same time, Mark took a position as office manager for a friend's growing firm. That income meant much more financial stability for our family, which we sorely needed. So, with Aleeta and Adam in school full time, I took over running the ad agency. Life was busy. The business was expanding, and so was I.

In order to fulfill my roles of wife, mother, and business owner, I would get up at four o'clock in the morning to finish up design projects and plan the busy day for my small staff. I didn't mind. I loved mornings. I sat doing what I enjoyed, with several pounds of M&Ms and Hershey's Assorted Minis to keep me company. It was a routine I looked forward to.

At least one day each week, I ordered a Subway delivery at my office and would, of course, treat the staff. Subway didn't normally deliver to home businesses, but I was such a good customer that they accommodated me. Besides the sandwiches for my staff, I always ordered three foot-long sandwiches, on the pretense of getting the extras for my husband or kids when they got home.

I don't think I fooled anyone. No one in my family ever saw those extra subs. But everyone could see what they were doing to me. And increasingly there were humiliating moments when my weight became the focal point of my world.

We used to go to a family camp in New Hampshire called Camp Spofford with our friends Dan and Cathy Getz and their family. They had two boys near Adam's age, two girls near Aleeta's age, and an older son. Cathy and I were best friends, and we did everything together, including dieting. One vacation I tried hard to be more active despite my excessive size. The kids had taken out paddle boats with Mark. Dan and their oldest son, Danny, were in a rowboat, and Cathy and I decided to follow in a canoe. I had spent every summer growing up on the water in Maine. Boating and swimming were second nature to me. This would be fun.

We were told we had to wear life preservers. One thing I did know was that I did not need a life preserver. Ever since I had reached three hundred pounds, I could float a foot above water without even treading water. No kidding! I just sat there and didn't move and didn't sink. I couldn't even swim to the bottom of the pool anymore because I was too buoyant. Cathy was the only one I ever told. She couldn't believe her eyes when I showed her in her backyard pool one day. I always made sure I looked like I was treading water when others were around and kept moving my arms and legs. So I didn't need a life preserver. It was impossible for me to drown, but I wasn't about to share that with the teens running the boat launch.

We each grabbed a life preserver, and Cathy put hers on. I found the largest one available and still couldn't buckle it up. No one was watching, so I tucked the straps in so they wouldn't dangle and hoped no one would say anything. I looked ridiculous with this orange ring around my twenty-two-inch neck.

Cathy got in the canoe, but I couldn't see much with the life preserver riding up so high on my weighty shoulders and upper body. I looked like a pimple about to pop. I couldn't see where I was going. I stepped gently into what I thought was the middle of the canoe and promptly tipped us over into the murky shallow waters. We both had on our beautiful new coverups and looked like a muddy mess.

The overly concerned teens came running to help the two fat ladies flailing in the shallow waters of the lake. We got up as quickly as we could, and good-naturedly Cathy agreed to try it again. I'd get it right this time. Sure enough, I flipped us a second time! I think even Cathy's calm, gentle demeanor was slightly ruffled.

Dan and Danny compassionately paddled over and offered to take us in the rowboat. It was much more stable. I looked at it and wondered if it was possible to flip that as well. I didn't think so. Everyone held their breath as I stepped in. The boat rode low in the water, but stayed stable.

We made it out to the "sunken island" where the snorkeling was best. I eased myself out of the boat, along with everyone else, without too much difficulty. The one thing I didn't foresee was having to get back in.

After thirty minutes of snorkeling it was time to head back. We were half a mile out. Dan and Danny and Cathy all pulled themselves into the boat. With my first attempt I knew I was in for trouble. The first to try to help me was Cathy while the guys busied themselves with the oars, pretending to be consumed with their tasks and not notice. Before long, all four of us were pulling and pushing. We all tried to hoist my body into that stupid rowboat. It just wasn't going to happen.

After about fifteen minutes we had only one option. Dan rowed back to shore and I held on to a line in the back of the boat as they towed me home. I'm not going to tell you how I felt or how it looked. It's enough that I've told you that it happened.

feeling the pain

My weight began to affect everything in my life, including how long it took to park the car (I would circle the lot for up to a half hour to find a spot close to the store entrance) and how we spent our family vacations (many more movies than bike rides). It reached out and choked every area of my world. I couldn't go horseback riding, though I shared my daughter's passion for it and watched her ride weekly for six years. I couldn't go on amusement park rides with my children because I couldn't fit into the seats.

The first time I realized this was when Aleeta and Adam were quite young. I waited in line with both of them and Mark for about twenty minutes to go on a large, flying swing ride. When the gate opened, we hurried to our swings. I grabbed one and pulled it behind me, but when I went to sit down, I was shocked and horrified to find that I couldn't get my butt into the chair! In complete humiliation, with a beet-red face and tears stinging my checks, I hastily made my way past everyone and out of the ride area. It had never occurred to me that I might not be able to fit, and I think I was in shock the rest of the day.

I began avoiding children who were likely to make comments about my size and rarely went to the children's section of the library even though I had two children.

In 1994, Mark and I went to Newport, RI where we rented scooters for the day. The rental clerk's comment: "You're obviously over the weight limit, but we'll rent to you if the tires hold out."

Once even my five-year-old niece sweetly asked why I was so big. It was so innocent, as though she were asking me to tell her my favorite color.

"Because I eat too much, dear."

"Why don't you stop eating so much, Auntie Kim?"

Out of the mouths of babes.

Sleeping was a nightmare all by itself. When I woke up in the middle of the night, I could never find a comfortable position again. My hips would fall asleep or my back would ache. And it took so much effort to turn from side to side, hoisting the bulk of my weight up and around. But staying in the same position was just as painful. Our bed was on the verge of breaking and complained loudly with every movement I made. *How I missed sleeping on my stomach!* I remembered the feeling of melting into my mattress, of being one with my bed. It was a delicious feeling I hadn't experienced in years.

And the snoring! My sleep apnea was so bad that sometimes I even woke myself up! I could really rock the house. It kept me from going on overnight field trips with my children. I felt self-conscious sleeping at family members' homes. I even hated falling asleep on a long car ride or on a vacation with other extended family members because I snored loudly as soon as I nodded off—and sometimes even before.

One time I shared a hotel room with Cathy and two other women from our church. I tried to stay awake until everyone else fell asleep, hoping that then my snoring would go unnoticed. It didn't work. One of the ladies, tired herself from the long day, had an awfully hard time with my snoring and kept waking me up with an increasingly annoyed "Kim!" In utter embarrassment, I lay there until I was certain everyone was asleep, then tiptoed out of the room into the hotel hallway.

My plan was to get another room (which I could ill afford) without anyone knowing and to sneak back into our shared room in the morning. Unfortunately, the hotel was booked solid, and there was a late-night wedding that filled the atrium with guests. I couldn't sleep in the car because I wasn't the one driving and I didn't have a key. So I wandered around the hotel until I found an empty sauna and lay down on the wooden bench. I had no pillow, no blanket, and a sense of dread that someone might walk in at any moment. Or maybe someone would call security after hearing me snore through those thick sauna walls and think I was an inebriated wedding guest who had lost her way.

I slept very little that night. Early the next morning, I cheerfully strolled back into our bedroom with a bucket of ice from down the hall. The girls were just getting up. They were none the wiser. No one ever knew except Cathy, in whom I confided the next day, and who wept for and with me.

what kind of wake-up call was i waiting for?

On August 18, 1991, our pastor, David McIntyre, preached a sermon on gluttony. He said it was one of the hardest sermons he had ever given; I felt it was one of his best. I got a tape of it and have listened to it many times in the years since. He talked about Yankee Stadium losing four thousand seats during its renovation in the 1990s because they had to add several inches to each seat to make room for expanding Americans. But then he really got my attention when he talked about how the Israelites in the Old Testament craved meat more than God.

I remember thinking, "Oh my gosh, how can that be? Who could love food more than God?" And then I realized, *that was me*! I mean, I really didn't . . . or did I? Where was my time spent, where was my focus, my enjoyment? I realized where my heart was. Food was my first love. And I didn't know how to change that.

what do you do when nothing fits?

As I got larger and larger, I lost interest in how I looked. My clothes became a source of frustration for me and everyone else in our household. I owned clothing in nearly every size from 16—now my dream clothes that I hadn't fit into in years—on up. They filled boxes in the attic and crammed my closet and drawers. I even took up space in everyone else's closets, though I wore only a small percentage of what I owned. There were probably only five or six outfits (most of them alike except for the color) that fit and looked good on me at any given time.

Worse still, I kept ruining the few clothes I *could* wear. I had to change my shirt frequently because I kept getting food stains across my chest and stomach. I weighed more than three hundred pounds. My napkin didn't cover much. I couldn't push in very far. Trying to bring food from the plate to my mouth meant traveling quite a distance—and even the most careful and slow eater (which I wasn't) was likely to suffer spills.

I wore shoes out quickly, too, no matter the cost or quality, so I shopped only at discount stores, knowing that whatever I bought would soon become worn and misshapen. I almost never wore socks—too much added bulk. I hated the way my feet and ankles looked as they spread over the sides of my shoes. Fortunately, I rarely saw them, anyway.

I could wear only slip-on shoes, and getting into socks or panty hose—when I did want to wear them—was nearly impossible. To get them on, I'd have to sit on my bed, hoist one leg up, and bend it as far as I could toward my body (which wasn't far at all, maybe halfway). To reach my feet, I took a deep breath and went at it. If it was a good day, my face turned only slightly purple as I struggled to get the item over my toes and pulled up into place.

Even jewelry became an issue. I'd wear a thin necklace (or none at all) and very small earrings. Sometimes I wore the same pair for months at a time. I didn't want anything to call attention to me or any part of my body. Most jewelry didn't fit me, anyway. Mark once bought me a beautiful scarab bracelet, and the jeweler had to add extra links. But probably the saddest day of all was when, after twelve years of marriage, my wedding bands had to be cut off. I had waited dangerously long to have them removed. It all but ruined them and I haven't worn one since.

ignoring the shame

You might think that one of these episodes would be the last straw, the final indignity that hurt so much or shook me so that I had to make some drastic change in my life. Unfortunately, that wasn't the case. As I got heavier and heavier, I had a difficult time looking professional. New clients weren't easy to come by. It was hard for people to notice my work and not me at first-time meetings. And my energy level was decreasing, along with my wardrobe.

One time I was directing a photo shoot for former Connecticut governor John Rowland. I had planned to wear a classic black-and-white houndstooth skirt. The skirt fit me well, so I always kept it in my closet, and I thought it would be perfect for the big day. But on the morning of the shoot, I grabbed the skirt and eased it down over my head to my waist, and was horrified to find that it wouldn't zip up. What had fit me so well only a month before wouldn't even close now. I panicked and hunted for a safety pin. Zipping the skirt halfway up, I put the pin below the zipper tongue so it wouldn't unzip. I figured that the jacket would cover it and all would be fine.

I looked in the mirror, which I usually avoided, and first noticed my face. It was so bloated, so distorted. I didn't even look like me anymore. My neck hung out almost as far as my face. I was disgusted. "Well, enjoy it," I said aloud. "This time next month you'll wish you looked *this* good." I knew it was true. I was still gaining weight daily.

Then I made myself look at the rest of my body. I noticed that the back of my skirt hem was eight inches higher than the front, which came down below my knees. I rolled up the front of the skirt waistband an inch or two.

There. Now it was even. The problem was, it had turned into a miniskirt. I looked ridiculous! I sucked in my stomach, zipped the skirt up further and placed an extra safety pin along the zipper. The hem of my skirt was much improved, but the waistband was digging into me terribly. I knew the pain would only worsen as the day went on. I prayed that the safety pins would hold for the next few hours!

That was the last time I wore that skirt for ten years.

The larger I got, the less I wanted to meet with clients. I hired a wonderful, energetic young woman named Sarah who was a fast learner and great with clients. I took fewer and fewer meetings, focused on the design and marketing work, and tried to take myself out of the public eye. But embarrassing situations still followed me.

We had a daily end-of-day pickup from Airborne Express, and we always left the packages in a drop box near the business entrance in our backyard. One day, I was rushing to pick up my kids from a friend's house after everyone had gone home. I ran out of the office and the door locked behind me. But in my haste I had caught a big chunk of my dress in the door. No matter how much I pulled and tugged, it would not give. I tried, but I couldn't manage to rip the strong flannel material.

My keys were in my car on the other side of the parking area, well out of my reach. I was stuck. Either I could wait several hours until someone came home, or I could slip out of my dress. I chose the latter. It wasn't easy, because such a large portion of the skirt was caught. I got down on my knees and began struggling to pull the dress off over my head. Getting this dress off was usually difficult; in this situation it was almost impossible. I weighed around three hundred pounds at the time. I struggled for quite a while, becoming more and more desperate.

I finally was able to get it up over my head, though my arms were still stuck behind me. As I knelt in my undergarments and strained to lift my head, my eyes locked with those of the Airborne Express man. He hadn't bothered turning his truck down into the driveway, but was ever so slowly driving past my driveway entrance, a horrified expression on his face.

I'm sure it wasn't a pretty sight. With the strength of ten men, I yanked my arms out of that dreadful dress and made a mad dash for my car. What I didn't anticipate was that my legs had fallen asleep and couldn't support me. I skidded on my knees and fell sideways on the icy pavement. My humiliation was complete.

Somehow I got into the car and huddled as low as I could go. I peered out over the dashboard just in time to see the driver's head duck back inside his truck. He revved the motor, drove on, and never returned. I grabbed my keys, ran back to open my office door, threw my dress on in one fell swoop, and raced back to my car to go get the kids. It wasn't until later that evening that I noticed my scraped-up knees.

You'd think this episode might have been my final wake-up call, but it wasn't. Then my beloved husband Mark, a type I diabetic since the age of seven, began to suffer health problems and had to be hospitalized for nearly three months. In the midst of caring for him, I realized that here I was with a perfectly healthy body that I was destroying, while my husband was fighting for his life against a disease he hadn't brought on himself. *What was I doing? Why was I so weak, so overwhelmed by this desire to eat?* Why did I have strength in so many areas of my life except this one?

I had no answer to my questions. And my life was about to get even more complicated. In 1999, when Aleeta was thirteen and Adam was eleven, our son Alan was born. Alan rocked our orderly world. He was not the quiet, twice-a-day napper that my first two had been. As adorable as he was, we needed all four sets of hands to keep him happy. My parents, who had moved back east to Massachusetts, helped when they could.

When Alan was just a year old, we left him for ten days with my mom and dad and took our older kids to Europe. We had been given free airfare through a student exchange program, and as big and uncomfortable as I was, as short on funds as we were, we decided we might never get a chance to travel like this again.

The four of us packed adventure after adventure into those ten short days. I'd wanted us to see so much, we rarely slept two nights in the same hotel. I had no idea the impact my size would have when I made the plans, and I suffered for it. Because we were on a very strict budget, we had precious little money for cab fares. Walking our modus operandi, but I could barely keep up.

I waited exhausted by the prison gates as my family inspected the crown jewels at the Tower of London. But worst of all was nearly getting stuck in the upper hallways of St. Paul's Cathedral in London. Aleeta and Adam were so enthralled with the ancient, small passageways and wanted us to see them. After trying to inch my way in, I was afraid I wouldn't be able to get back out. *I simply couldn't fit.* By the time we finished touring five countries in ten days, I was a wreck. The only things that kept me going were the crepes in France and the fresh scones in London!

food, food, it's all about the food

By this time my life was completely centered on food, and I was dragging my family along with me. Holidays, vacations, even our weekly Friday family movie night—everything focused on what we were going to eat. At the end of each week, I'd take the kids to rent a movie and then to the grocery store to pick out everyone's favorite choices for "snack dinner." We filled the cart with pizza bagels, potato skins, Cheez Whiz, summer sausage meat sticks, crackers, chips and dip, little hot dogs wrapped up in croissants and, of course, an assortment of desserts.

And the candy—every holiday had its own selection in the stores. As soon as the Christmas candy vanished it was time to stock up for Valentine's Day and then Easter. I loved Halloween candy best of all. I couldn't wait to run out and buy a supply of it when it first appeared on retail shelves in August. I replenished it dozens of times before October 31— even though I knew that, because of the narrow country road we lived on, we'd had only three trick-or-treaters in the twenty years we lived there!

Even though I regularly ate large meals at home, my frequent between-meal snacks added some serious pounds. I would go to our local Duchess drive-through several times a week and order my "regular": two hot dogs with the works, a double cheeseburger with the works, two fries, two German chocolate cake slices, and two diet sodas. (I thought if I ordered two sodas the person taking the order would think it was for two. I don't think I ever fooled anyone.)

And I couldn't go to a drive-through with a car full of hungry kids and not buy something for them as well. Not only were these between-meal "snacks" murder on our checking account, but I was literally poisoning my own children, feeding them so much unhealthy food, and more important, teaching them unhealthy eating habits. Even though I knew what I was doing was wrong for me and for them, I just couldn't stop. I was like a junkie, addicted to food.

That's not to say I didn't still "try" the new diets when they came out. But the time I lasted on them became shorter and shorter. My weight fluctuations were huge now. I could lose eight pounds in one week, but I could gain that much back and more in just a few days. It became increasingly difficult to stick to a diet for any time at all.

Once, while weighing close to 320 pounds, I went to a nearby shopping center to run some errands. Although I had been doing fairly well on my latest diet, I allowed the aromas from the local bakery to lure me inside. I quickly ordered my favorite, a nine-inch double layer cake.

A wave of excitement came over me. My diet was over—I could eat! I'd blown it. My elation was quickly followed by a wave of sadness. It was over . . . and I was still trapped. Trapped in this body behind enemy lines in a prison I couldn't escape.

I was quickly brought back to the present by the salesgirl. "What?"

"Do you want anything written on your cake?" she asked. I hesitated only for a moment. "Why don't you write 'Congratulations Kimberly' on it," I answered, feeling complete disgust with myself. She did and brought it out for my inspection.

I hurried out to the car with my purchases and ate the entire cake sitting in the front seat. I cried all the way home.

Everyday life continued to be filled with humiliation and angst. In parking lots I frequently cleaned off my car and the ones next to mine with my stomach and my rear end, trying to get in and out. I outgrew many plus-size clothing stores and could find clothes to fit me in only a few specialty shops.

My mom and I went out hunting for some new pants one afternoon. I hated shopping now! I told Mom to look for a size 34. "I don't understand that size. Is it European?" she asked. "No, Mom. You just start at 16 and keep counting: 16, 18, 20, 22, until you get all the way up to 34. It's definitely American, just fat." We found a pair of lightweight blue capris.

They were the largest size in the store. What was I going to do when I outgrew those?

I soon lost the ability to stick to a diet at all. Most home scales go up to only three hundred pounds, so I don't even know what I weighed at that point. At doctor's visits, my weight was listed as OTC—off the charts.

running out of time

Our last child, Andrew, was born in February 2001, and shortly after that Mark and I let our staff go. As my weight was increasing, my self-confidence was decreasing. So when clients moved on, I never replaced them and eventually went from a bustling small agency with an "Employer of the Year" award to an independent freelance designer with a handful of projects.

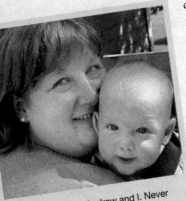
Six-month-old Andrew and I. Never thought I'd be around to see him grow up.

In those years after the births of the boys, my quality of life went downhill dramatically. Walking was difficult, breathing a constant chore. I tried to do everything I could possibly do upstairs before coming downstairs. If it meant carrying enormous loads, I'd do that, rather than go up and down. Whenever I could, I asked my teenagers to run errands for me, even around my own house.

I experienced some health scares. After I had heart palpitations, the doctors made me wear a twenty-four-hour heart monitor, but they found nothing seriously wrong—except my excessive weight. A few years later, I ruptured a disk in my back. I actually lost weight because I was in too much agony to get up and cook anything. I couldn't drive for several months, so my access to fast food was limited, too. But the weight loss was temporary, once my back healed.

Then, in 2000, I broke out in terrible sores all over my body. I was diagnosed with vasculitis, and it was just awful. I was nearing 350 pounds, covered in oozing boils, and I could hardly walk. It was midsummer and the medication—prednisone—caused me to retain fluid. I was miserable.

That was the same time we had a huge family reunion to celebrate my grandfather's eightieth birthday. More than a hundred family members were coming, some of whom I hadn't seen since I was a child. *So this was how everyone would remember me.* Not only did I not lose weight for the occasion, I spent most of the day "help-ing" in the kitchen and cleaned up the remainder of the enormous sheet cake after everyone had gone home.

I was despondent.

Every time I answered the phone I was painfully aware of my heavy breathing and would often make an excuse of having just "run" to the phone, even though I hadn't even gotten out of my chair.

At the mall, I could walk for only a few hundred feet and then I'd have to sit on a bench and catch my breath. Every time I stood up, it would

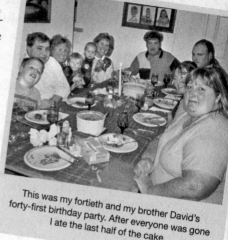

This was my fortieth and my brother David's forty-first birthday party. After everyone was gone I ate the last half of the cake.

take a minute or two for the pain in my feet to go away. I was ex-hausted all the time. By my fortieth birthday, I was nearly 350 pounds. It hurt standing up. It hurt sitting down. It hurt lying down. I just plain hurt. Inside and out.

I remember one morning walking down the stairs and saying to my-self, "Don't eat for ten minutes. After that, you can eat anything and every-thing you can find. Just don't eat for ten minutes."

I couldn't do it. I walked into the kitchen and began eating.

I didn't even feel desperate any more. I was numb. I completely gave up and vowed I would never diet again. For nearly a year I didn't.

I really *was* eating myself to death. Difficult as it is to admit, I was so hopeless at this point. I, the queen of dieting, could no longer stick to a diet for even half a day. I was completely out of control. When I wasn't eating, which wasn't very often, I was thinking about food, buying food, or planning what to eat.

I knew there was no way I would ever lose the weight now. Even if I could (by some miracle) stick to a diet for eight weeks, and even if I managed to lose five pounds each week, I would still be wearing the same ginormous stretch pants, I would still be more than three hundred pounds, and no one would notice the loss except me.

It was hard to understand how I'd gotten where I was. I had a hus-band who loved me, four wonderful children, a lovely home, and work I enjoyed. I had been so blessed, and yet I was throwing it all away.

Somewhere inside, I think I always hoped someone would see the

my story

27

severity of my plight, see my desperate need and find a way to help me. I believe I wanted *someone* or *something* to intervene, to put restrictions on me, somehow take the decision making out of my hands, removing my ability to overeat.

That's what appealed so much to me about gastric bypass.

When my kids were growing up, they took martial arts classes several days each week. The moms and dads would sit or stand around and chat while watching the class. Debbie, one of the moms, was about my size at the time. She was a little younger than I was and very pretty. We talked about diets together over the years; neither of us had ever succeeded.

Then one day I saw her at a basketball game. Aleeta and Adam had stopped taking karate, so it had been almost a year since I had seen Debbie. She was thin and she was gorgeous.

I just stared and stared. Finally I got up the nerve to approach her. My weight during the year had gone in the opposite direction and I felt fatter than ever. I didn't even waste time with small talk. I couldn't. "Debbie, you look fabulous! How did you do it?" We spent a half an hour talking about her decision to have bypass surgery. She felt wonderful, she said, and she looked wonderful.

She had gotten to her goal weight after the operation. She also said she had recently put a few pounds back on. She said she wished it were still like it had been in the beginning, right after the surgery before she could eat very much, when the choice to overeat was out of her hands. Now she could eat more and was afraid her eating was getting off track.

All I could see was her thin ankles.

All I could hear was how good it felt.

How I wanted that surgery! Then she told me the costs involved, and I knew it would be impossible for me. But if I'd had the money at that moment, I would have driven right over to the hospital, lain down on a table, and asked them to do the surgery right then! I envied Debbie more than anyone in the world. But surgery was an impossibility for me. *I was on my own.*

trying *again*!

the turning point

I'd always loved the quiet of mornings, getting up early before everyone else and spending time alone. With a lively eight-month-old, an overactive toddler, and two busy teenagers, this was the one time I had the house to myself.

One morning early in October 2001, everything changed. I walked into the kitchen and bypassed the cupboards and refrigerator. I headed directly to the table and laid my worn-out Bible on it. I opened up to Psalm 121: "I will lift up mine eyes unto the hills, from whence cometh my help. My help cometh even from the Lord . . ."

I read it again. I closed my eyes and sat quietly. I remembered the words of Pastor Dave from nearly a decade ago, about how the people had loved food more than God. I prayed a little. Emotions flooded me like the sunlight streaming in on me through the double windows to where I was sitting.

I was tired. Tired of living at this size. Tired of fighting. Fighting my weight, fighting ambivalence toward food, fighting with my clothes and food budget and shortness of breath. I hated living in this body. I wanted out. I wanted . . .

What did I want? *Peace.*

My feet hurt, my back hurt, and I was always uncomfortable. I was so tired. Sick and tired. And as afraid as I was of giving up overeating, of giving up eating as much as I wanted, whatever I wanted, I was more afraid of not giving it up.

But how? What should I do? I started praying. But the words weren't coming. I didn't know what to say. I had said it all before. *Millions of times.* That day it was more than a prayer. It was a groaning too deep for words—short, simple, deep.

"God, I need help. I've really made a mess of things and somehow, as much as I love you and adore my family, somehow I've put eating above everything else in my life. I'm sorry. I want to change, but I don't know how. I really don't think I can."

I almost said "Amen" at this point, but then a lightbulb came on.

I couldn't change my heart, but I really believed God could.

"God? I've prayed so many times before. I've tried so many times. I know I can't do this, but God, I believe *you* can. Help me, God. Please help me change my heart and my priorities and . . . my life."

At the end of my brief prayer, I felt lighter. I sat there, still. The baby was awake and calling me. But I felt a peace, as if a burden had been lifted from me. I hadn't prayed expecting change. I didn't expect anything. It was just a simple, honest outpouring of my broken heart.

I went on with my day as usual and didn't think about it again. Somewhere, though, deep down inside, was the realization that I had been given the strength to try again.

That was the miracle. After months of ignoring the pain and the problem. After years of hoping to be rescued. After a lifetime of putting food above everything else in my life. *I was ready to make a change.*

getting started

The next day I saw my girlfriend Cathy. She was walking toward my car in her driveway, and I nearly accused her: "You've lost weight!"

"How can you tell?" she asked. "No one else has noticed. I've only lost four pounds!" But I knew. *I knew.* I could practically smell it.

"I started Weight Watchers again," she went on, "and I didn't want to tell you because I've no idea if it's going to 'work,' but it feels different this time."

"Can I come?" I pleaded.

"Of course. Thursdays at twelve thirty."

"I'll be there," I said. And I was.

I, who months earlier had given up on ever dieting again, joined Weight Watchers—one more time—on October 4, 2001, and weighed in at 347 pounds. But even seeing the numbers themselves couldn't squelch the eagerness I felt to be back again. I was finally ready.

I embraced the Weight Watchers Points program immediately. We were a perfect fit. It wasn't the first time I had tried it, but it was the first time I put everything I had into it. A definite learning curve was involved. It took a lot of effort in the beginning to learn the values of all the foods and how to plan what I was going to eat. There was a lot more to it than just *how much food* I could have, there was also *what kind of food*. So much in each category: fruits, vegetables, protein, fat, carbs and water. Each day had to be well balanced as well as the right number of points (calories, fat, and fiber). It was a real commitment, but for some reason I was excited to get going.

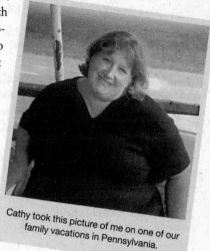

Cathy took this picture of me on one of our family vacations in Pennsylvania.

I didn't tell anyone except Cathy, Mark, and my kids that I was starting something new. I had started so many times before and stopped that I just didn't want anyone knowing right away. Besides, I thought it would be fun to surprise everyone, especially my parents, who were so concerned for my health.

But surprising my parents was not to be.

Three days after this major turning point in my life, my wonderful, beloved father had a heart attack and died the next day. He never knew that his prayers for his little girl had finally been answered.

In the midst of deep grief, without much practice in using the Points program—and surrounded by an overwhelming quantity of catered food and other people's cooking—I did my best to stay with it. I don't know why. I didn't care very much at that point, and no one even knew I was dieting.

I kept telling myself that it would have been so easy to put it off for another time. *No one would blame me. With all the stress and grief, who would expect me to keep dieting? The timing just wasn't right, right?*

But something inside me *had* changed, and I stuck with it.

coping with grief

In the days that followed, we traveled to Massachusetts, to Maine, and back home to Connecticut. We drove for hours. We ate out. I kept quietly working at it. Nearly a week later, early on the morning of my father's memorial service, with a house full of extended family and catered food, I crept down the stairs. Homemade pies, cakes, and bread, sent by caring friends and church members, were on the table and counters. Casseroles and salads lined the fridge. It was too much. I planned on eating everything in sight! I was tired of trying to figure out Points and I was hungry. Who could blame me for giving up after all this? I was ready to binge.

I walked toward the table, plate in hand. The first dish I reached for was an apple crisp, nestled in among all the other goodies. There was a note on top: "Low-Fat Apple Crisp: only two points per cup."

I don't even know how it got there or where it came from, but that little reminder was all I needed to keep going. I had two cups of it with my coffee and I was ready to face the day. I never looked back again after that moment.

Two weeks later I returned to Weight Watchers—and I'd lost more than seven pounds. That was just the beginning. I often wonder—if I *had* given up right after my father died, would I have ever gone back? Where would I be now?

Life settled into a routine. Every Thursday the boys and I would pick up Cathy and we'd head to our weekly meeting. God bless Cathy. I couldn't have done it without her. My strong-willed Alan was 2½ years old, and Andrew was nine months, so I sometimes felt like I was raising them at those Thursday meetings. Cathy and I became friends with our regular meeting buddies, especially our wonderful leader, Beth. Sometimes I got only the beginning and the end of her talk because I was potty-training Alan and glued to the bathroom in the back of the room. Other times, I felt like all I did for the entire thirty minutes was breast-feed Andrew. Try running around after a three-year-old with another child attached to you. You get the picture!

It would have been nice to sit there and really listen and participate wholeheartedly. But there were always drink spills, food messes, diaper explosions, and more than a few temper tantrums.

Was it worth it? You bet it was!

And I was so grateful for the support of the other members. It was a noon meeting—right around the lunch hour. But even when I brought Burger King kids' meals with me for my boys, no one ever complained about the odors of chicken nuggets and French fries wafting through the air!

On non-meeting days, Cathy and I would frequently meet at Ruby

Tuesday for lunch. We'd bring our plan books and figure out together what we could eat. There was so much on the menu we could fit into our program, we both could scarcely believe it. Every week we'd ask each other the same question, "It's been another whole week . . . do you really think it will last?"

To paraphrase what it says in Proverbs 27:17, "As iron sharpens iron, so one friend sharpens another." And we did.

three cheers!

We hardly noticed as the weeks flew by. I was so excited for Cathy, as was everyone in the Thursday noon meeting. She had started in September and had continued to lose steadily until she reached her goal in the spring of 2002. Nine months and eighty-five pounds later, she was done. But she continued going to meetings to support me.

For me, obviously, the journey took longer. After several months of following the program, I had lost thirty-five pounds, but it wasn't really noticeable. I was still wearing those same stretch pants and I still wasn't yet under three hundred pounds. There were days when, despite my excitement and gratitude, I became impatient and discouraged. Was it going to "keep working"? Could I really get down to a size 22/24 (my goal at the time)? I kept plugging away. Yet in the back of my mind was this nagging fear that at any moment the bubble could pop and I might find myself out of control, eating as I used to, with the numbers on the scale climbing back up. I dared not hope. I really worked at controlling my thoughts. No more daydreaming about the goodies in the bakery. If a thought popped into my mind about eating something I hadn't planned on, I shut it down as fast as I could. No more mental anguish. Dealing with desires became so much easier.

My family was always there to support me. Aleeta took a picture of me one or two Thursdays each month in my "weigh-in outfit." I always wore the same clothes so that I would know exactly how much my weight was. (That's how the progression photos on the back cover came to be.) The pictures provided steady evidence that my body was changing, and I could easily look back to see how far I'd come.

Adam always had an encouraging word, and I smiled when his friends told me how "hot you're looking, Mrs. B!" The whole family cheerfully tried every new recipe I concocted. They didn't always like them (neither did I), but at least they were willing to try.

Each week after weighing in I'd get in the car and call Mark, then my mom and then my sister, Heather, who cheered with me on the good weeks and offered a word of encouragement on the rough ones. They all had so much faith in me, and I clung to that when mine wavered.

As the months passed, I became an expert at converting my recipes to healthier versions, and I got great at finding grocery items that were low in points and yummy. I was still a volume eater, but now the calories were within my daily range.

At last, I was under three hundred pounds. I felt like a beauty queen. Imagine feeling like a beauty queen at 290 pounds! And as spring turned to summer, seven or eight months after I started, people began noticing.

When I went to my church's Memorial Day picnic, I brought my own low-fat hot dogs to grill. The guys threw them on with a grin as I threatened their lives if they mixed them up with the high-fat ones. I had learned that being prepared added up to weight loss on the scale, so I brought a lot of my own food wherever I went. No one seemed to notice or care, something I used to be self-conscious about. Not anymore. As a matter of fact, several people commented that they wished they had done the same thing.

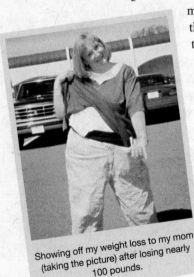

Showing off my weight loss to my mom (taking the picture) after losing nearly 100 pounds.

The more I put into my weeks' food planning and preparation, the more pounds I lost. "If you bite it, write it," became my motto. I never put anything in my mouth that I hadn't planned out. The hard work paid off.

When I hit my one-year anniversary I weighed in at 224 pounds. I was a size 20 and felt wonderful. My "diet" was finally becoming my lifestyle.

About this time the unexpected happened. I found a lump. I knew I should tell Mark, see a doctor, something, but I didn't. I waited, checking it frequently, hoping and praying it would go away. It didn't. As a matter of fact, it seemed to grow larger daily. I could put off telling him no longer. Where do you begin? How do you tell someone you love that you found a lump? It seemed particularly cruel now—just as I was losing so much weight and getting healthier. I had lost more than a hundred pounds, but I still had a hundred to go. I so wanted to see this thing through to the end, but now . . .

I lay in bed on my back watching him get ready for work, "Mark," I began. He turned around quickly at the tone of my voice. I hurried on, trying to keep it light. "I have a lump. It's right here on my side. It was so small just a few months ago, but it's gotten larger so quickly. I know I should have said something sooner." My voice trailed off.

"Let me see." He came over, and I guided his hand to the area. He felt it carefully. His tenderness brought tears to my eyes. A puzzled expression crossed his face as he kept probing. Then a smile. Even a chuckle. "How long have you waited to tell me this?" he asked. "Several weeks," I answered. "What . . ."

He stood up smiling. "I think, Mrs. Bensen, you'll find a lump on the other side as well. It's your hip bone, Kim. You just haven't felt it in so long, you've forgotten what it feels like."

It took a minute for it to sink in. I furiously felt both sides and the realization that he was right washed over me. I was fine! That awful heaviness I had been carrying immediately lifted. I don't know if I laughed or cried more that morning, but I remember thinking this would be a great story if I ever found the courage to tell it. How embarrassing, but how funny!

Of course, there were struggles along the way. I hit my first plateau. I hit my second plateau. Try sticking to your diet perfectly for four weeks and not losing a pound. What could be more discouraging? The bigger weight losses just weren't happening any more. I was frustrated, and my determination was waning. For the first time I didn't call my mother or sister after my meeting to tell them how I had done. *Why bother?* I thought. On my way to the front seat, my phone rang. "How'd you do this week?" It was Heather.

"I *did* great, but you'd never know it by the scales. I was just thinking of having a meatball sub with cheese for lunch instead of a turkey and veggie." There was a pause. I didn't even have to say how discouraged I was. She knew.

"Hey, sis," Heather said, "I'd say have the meatball, but . . . don't you actually like the turkey and veggie better?!" She was right. I wanted the meatball only because I was mad and it was high in fat, not because I actually preferred it. How stupid!

We started laughing together. One of us snorted and we laughed harder. I felt lighter than I had in weeks. She was right, the little brat! I had worked so hard at finding foods that I loved, it would be completely stupid to go on a binge now. The realization that I had finally found a way of eating that I enjoyed was very encouraging and just what I needed at that moment.

my story

Not long after that, Cathy and I were sitting in a meeting and a new woman joined the group. As usual, Beth announced weight losses and gave out awards. When she mentioned that I had lost 150 pounds, this woman was shocked and said, "Oh my gosh! I can't believe how much you've lost and how long you've been at it. I bet you can't wait until it's over!"

At first I didn't realize what she was talking about. Until *what* was over? Then it dawned on me. "Oh, I get it. When my diet's over! I used to think that way, too!" I told her. "But it'll *never* be over. The day I stop counting points is the day I'll start gaining weight again. And I like how I'm living. Why would I ever want to stop?"

I knew right then that I'd get there, however long it took. My original goal of getting to a size 22/24 had long since been achieved. Reaching my goal weight didn't seem impossible any longer. So I kept working and eventually broke through the two hundreds into the one hundreds (from Two-terville into One-derland, as we like to call it), which I hadn't seen since shortly after I was married. Next I hit 173½ pounds—I weighed as much as I had lost!

changing how i thought about food

For most of my life, I hated anything low fat. If I knew something was made with low-fat mayonnaise, forget it. I wouldn't even try it. (Right, Mom?) And believe me, I could tell. But as I lost weight and needed to satisfy myself with fewer calories, I knew that I should try lighter products. I taste-tested light dressings and enjoyed many of them; one week I decided to give low-fat mayonnaise a chance—and thought, this is good! Cathy and I continued going to Ruby Tuesday each week, but our orders changed to plain baked potatoes with sides of broccoli, hold the butter and oil. And we loved it!

"If I could have looked into the future and seen what I'd be ordering at Ruby Tuesday for lunch back when I started," I said once to Cathy, "I'd probably have quit right away." But this wasn't the deprivation I had once feared.

Along with my taste buds, my sizes were changing rapidly and, even though it would have been fun to hit the mall, it wouldn't have been worth the money. Instead, I shopped in my own closet—I had clothes in just about every size. Cathy gave me her hand-me-downs, and I also picked up a few things at thrift stores and consignment shops.

Finally, after all those weeks and months, the end was in sight.

The last few months were like clawing off the pounds. At the end of the summer of 2003, our family went back to Camp Spofford for a week-long vacation. There I started walking. It was the first aerobic exercise I'd done in years. Only months before, I had been unable to walk for five minutes without gasping for breath. Now I could move quickly and feel good every step of the way!

I really enjoyed my fast walks each morning. On the third day of vacation, I noticed that they had a triathlon coming up on Thursday—a combination of swimming, biking, and jogging. I decided that if I could find a bike, I'd enter.

I asked around and was able to borrow an old three-speed bike from someone's mother. I put my name on the list. Some people had signed up as teams; others were planning to do all three parts, as I was.

At one o'clock on Thursday, I stood on the beach with all the other participants. I was planning to take my time and just finish, but as I stood with all the others, their competitive spirit rubbed off on me. *I can swim pretty well, can't I?*

I decided to give it my all! The whistle blew and I charged, racing across the sand and high-stepping my way into the lake water. But something was wrong—every step with my right leg was agony. *What have I done?* Then I realized that with my first step I had pulled a muscle in my thigh. *What an idiot!*

I had to pull my leg along to continue. Everyone in the camp was watching. I wasn't going to quit. My fellow triathletes were getting farther and farther ahead of me, and I was still in ankle-deep water! *How humiliating.* Everyone was cheering, and my own group was screaming my name. *Kim! Kim! Go on, Kim! Run, Kim!* I looked like I was hunting seashells!

I finally made it out far enough and plunged underneath. Once I was swimming, the leg didn't hurt nearly as much. I actually made some headway. But I was still the last one to finish the swim. The spotters in the rowboats had nothing better to do in the end than hover near me. Everyone else was out of the water and on their bikes. As I started walking out of the water again (a *very* long, slowly sloping shallow section on this lake), the pain returned. The bikers had all left, and the attention of the entire beach was on my Sunday stroll out of the lake. I was too far away to tell anyone what had happened. I didn't want to sound like a poor sport, but it was awfully embarrassing to move that slowly without anyone knowing why.

I finally made it to shore and "ran" across the beach to the road. My husband knew something was wrong and encouraged me to stop, but I wanted to finish. *I needed to finish.* I doused my feet with water, slipped some sneakers on my wet feet, grabbed a T-shirt, hopped on my three-speed bike, and pedaled off after everyone else. They had already reached the top of the hill, turned the corner, and sped out of sight. Then I realized that I hadn't been on a bike since high school.

They say you never forget how to ride a bike. Well, for the first quarter of a mile I wondered if that was true. I was all over the road. And there was a huge hill. Even the lowest gear of this three-speed wasn't low enough! I did most of the work with my left leg (which probably explains why I was all over the road). I couldn't wait to be up that hill and out of sight of everyone in the camp. I could have *walked* faster, but I refused to get off and push.

Once I turned the corner I realized that I wasn't sure where I was going. I pulled the map out of my bathing suit. Mark had handed it to me with my T-shirt. It was pretty blurry and difficult to read. I was on a major road-way for this section and was honked at more than once. (And I'm sure it wasn't because I looked so good on that bike!) I continued on and finally turned off onto a quiet road. *More hills!* How could I end up in the same place and only pedal uphill the whole way? At least, that was how it seemed!

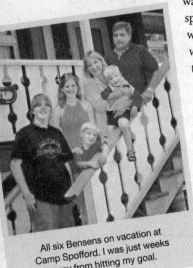

All six Bensens on vacation at Camp Spofford. I was just weeks away from hitting my goal.

Forty-five minutes later, I heard a car coming up beside me. It was Mark—just checking to make sure I was okay. As he drove slowly along-side me, I told him what I had done to my leg. He gave me a water bottle and some aspirin and left. It was nice to be loved!

By the end of the five miles I saw some people jogging back toward me, and I realized they were already halfway into their last leg of the triathlon. I waved and yelled, "Looking good!" as I passed them.

I finally made it around the lake. Two down, one to go.

I dropped my bike and started back in the direction I had just come from. Everyone was still there cheering as I jogged out of sight. Most of the way, I had to walk. My leg wasn't any worse, but I couldn't lift it at all. I kept going, but it was a slow shuffle. Everyone passed me and smiled. I actually enjoyed the solitude of the beautiful countryside and was pleased with myself despite my poor finish. In the end, the winner of the race jogged back to make sure I was all right.

I did finally finish, more than an hour after everyone else. A large crowd of supporters was still waiting for the last participant—me—and cheered as loudly as though I had finished first. I found out later that the written record of my results will forever be posted on their triathlon bulletin board. *Had I only known!*

from one goal to another

Finishing the triathlon felt really good, but my eyes were on another goal, one I had dreamed about forever. The only question was, *when* would I get there?

The top of the weight range given to me by Weight Watchers was 155 pounds. Once I hit that goal, I had to stay under that number for six weeks to receive the coveted Lifetime Membership award. The day finally came. After almost two years of hard work, planning, counting points, and attending meetings, I finally hit goal in mid-September. I called my mom and she cried. I called my sister and she screamed. She booked her flight from Minnesota for six weeks hence.

I looked at the calendar and realized that the day I would get my lifetime membership from Weight Watchers would be October 2—exactly two years from the day I first walked through those doors. My grandparents Bick and Marlene Stevens (Lifetime Members themselves) made plans to drive down from Maine. Mark and my brother, David, got the day off from work. All of my children and my mother would be there, as well as several friends. The only one who would be missing would be my dad. He would have been so proud!

I had decided to set a personal goal of losing an additional eight pounds below the top of the range. I wanted to weigh 147 pounds. I wanted to hit the big "two hundred pounds lost" on that same day, if possible.

With that goal in mind, I watched everything that went in my mouth, but the last four pounds just weren't coming off. Then, for about ten days I started gaining a pound every few days and couldn't figure out why. My weight climbed higher and higher. I could see not losing, but gaining? It just didn't make sense!

The day of my big weigh-in was drawing closer. Forget reaching my two-hundred-pound mark—now I was worried about even being able to stay within my range for my Lifetime Membership. I was climbing closer and closer back to 155 pounds. My sister's flight was booked, and everyone was planning to be there. How disappointing. How embarrassing it would be. What was going on here?

I spoke with Beth. We reviewed my diet, and she decided it might be water weight due to salt from the packaged turkey breast that I had added to my diet. I had been trying to increase my protein. She suggested I start eating lots of asparagus and drinking lemon tea—both natural diuretics.

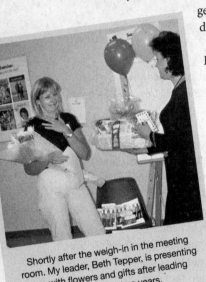

Shortly after the weigh-in in the meeting room. My leader, Beth Tepper, is presenting me with flowers and gifts after leading me to goal for two years.

I thought, "You've gotta be kidding me." But I was ready to give anything a try. Well, she was right. I'll spare you the details, but the asparagus appeared to be working.

Three days before the big weigh-in, the batteries in my scale wore out, and my darling daughter, Aleeta, dared me not to replace them. I took her up on her challenge.

My family arrived. We all headed for Weight Watchers the morning of October 2. We walked up to the front door of the building. There were signs everywhere. "BIGGEST LOSER KIM BENSEN. SHE LOST MORE THAN 200 LBS!" Speakers were blasting "Isn't She Lovely?" from inside the building. There were banners and balloons, flowers and so many people. Weight Watchers regional managers were in attendance, thirty people were waiting for me to weigh in—and I didn't have any idea what I weighed! *I could have strangled Aleeta.*

I was shaking as I stepped on the scale. Cameras were flashing. There was a new girl behind the counter who took forever reviewing my book. She didn't appear to comprehend the numbers. She looked at my book, back to the scale, back to my book. She said nothing. She'd be great at poker, I thought.

"Don't tell me if I'm over," I quipped nervously.

Silence.

I smiled through clenched teeth. "Tell me something. Anything."

Still nothing. Then, "Wow, you weigh one hundred forty-one pounds—

for a total of two hundred six pounds lost!" I had a meltdown right there on the scale.

Nearly blinded by flashbulbs, I stepped down off the scale into Mark's arms. My weight loss journey was finally over. Oh, I'd have to learn maintenance, and I'd still have future struggles, but I'd fought the fight. I finished the race. This was how it felt to reach the finish line.

I was *finally thin*!

to be continued . . .

Losing more than 200 pounds made a huge difference in my life. I can't even count all the ways, but here are a few of them:

I completely stopped snoring. No more sleep apnea.

I can cross my legs—oh, how I waited for that one!

I wear socks again, and I love to accessorize. (My daughter makes sure of it!)

I can walk into a room unnoticed.

I no longer need to create a mental map around tables and chairs to cross to the other side of a restaurant.

I don't think twice about the size of chairs before sitting in them, and, if one breaks, I can be sure it was the chair and not me at fault.

I can finally buckle up in the car or on an airplane.

And amusement park rides—I'm there!

I got a suntan for the first time in years.

I wear over-the-counter jewelry without extenders.

I have more energy than my four children—and that's saying a lot.

I no longer dread or fear doctor appointments.

All in all, I lost 212 pounds, lowered my cholesterol more than 200 points, lost oodles of inches—including 1½ inches in each wrist and 9 inches in my neck! I've gone down at least fourteen sizes, from a 6X to a size 6. I even lost one and a half shoe sizes (plus, I went from wide to normal widths) and four ring sizes. My feet, knees, and back never hurt any more (except after playing tackle football with my kids). I walk and do twenty push-ups and one hundred crunches every morning. I feel better, healthier, and look younger today than I did ten years ago.

Many wonderful things have happened since I stepped off that scale. Weight Watchers invited me to New York City for a makeover and to be a success story on their Web site, and I found out what it's like to be a star for a day. Then, a few months later a writer from *People* magazine saw my story and asked to feature me in the new magazine, *Your Diet*—and there I was, the subject of a two-page spread. That led to a January 2006 cover story in *Woman's World*.

Next came *Prevention* magazine. I'll never forget the day I received an advance copy of the issue in the mail. I opened the package carefully. The magazine was wrapped in individual tearsheets of the story. I held the packet tightly and paced the driveway as I read the article to Mark over the phone. The photo of the two of us was wonderful. I thought I couldn't have been more thrilled—until the actual magazine fell out from between the folds of the article. *There I was.* Staring back from the cover of *Prevention* magazine. *Me.* I couldn't believe it! I screamed and nearly scared my husband to death.

"I'm on the cover! Aaaaah!"

I thought it couldn't get any better, but later that week the *Today* show called. The producer asked, "Are you the Kim Bensen from the cover of *Prevention* magazine? Will you come share your story live on our show?"

Would I? As nervous as I was about appearing on national television, I knew I needed to do this—for me, for others. I remembered how important hearing success stories had been as I looked for ways to kick-start my own weight loss program. Since then I've been on the *Today* show several times, *Dr. Oz, Fox & Friends, ExtraTV,* and others. Sometimes I share my story and other times I cook. It's one of the highlights of my new life.

The response from America to my story was overwhelming. E-mails, phone calls, handwritten letters—all asking for details. What recipes did I use, and did I have any tips to share? How did I stay motivated for so long? And the most asked question, "What about all the loose skin?!" I

> Just remember . . . the only way
> you'll *never* lose weight is if you stop trying.

began spending up to several hours a day giving tips and emotional support to people I'd never met. But they weren't strangers, they were fellow strugglers fighting a common battle. I just wished it didn't take so long to repeat myself to each individual person.

Somewhere amidst the busyness of life we launched www.kimbensen. com and started sending out a regular e-newsletter. This helped me share information on a widespread basis, but it also brought more people to my Web site. And we found other ways to share recipes. One of the writers for *Woman's World* magazine suggested I put my recipes into a book. *Kim's Cookbooklet* was self-published first, and then came *Kim's Cookbooklet, Second Helping.*

I loved what I was doing! My online friendships were growing and my television opportunities were, too. I was still waitressing and Mark was still working full-time, but we began to dream about working together someday. Then, one month after being featured in *Prevention* magazine, something happened that brought my world crashing down around me.

life's changes

"This is Kim," I answered my cell as I always do when I'm in a hurry, without thinking or looking at the number.

I was on my way to the Weight Watchers center in Stratford, Connecticut, for my Monday night meeting. I still couldn't believe I was a Weight Watchers leader. After twenty years of struggling with hundreds and hundreds of pounds, I still expected to look in the mirror and see a 6X body staring back. But life was different now; life was good. I loved my job, my husband, and our four children. But after a weekend away to celebrate our twentieth wedding anniversary, I was running late, and Mark hadn't been feeling well all weekend. I was worried and distracted.

"Kim!" I didn't recognize the voice on the other end of the line.

"Who is this?"

"Kim, this is Dr. Farens."

"Hey!! Did you see Mark? He . . . wait . . . why are *you* calling me?

What's wrong, Dr. Farens?" My stomach sank. And my breath. I couldn't catch my breath.

"Kim, I need you to meet me at the hospital. Mark is either having a heart attack or has already had one."

"What?!" My world started to reel. I didn't understand what he was saying. Needless to say, I never made it to my meeting that night.

Mark survived his "significant" heart attack but had to have three surgeries implanting seven stents. This was the beginning of the end of our typical middle-class American life as we had known it.

Eight weeks after the heart attack, just as Mark was struggling to go back to work, he lost his job of thirteen years.

Mark had always been our sole income provider, except for my few cookbook sales and my two nights of waitressing each week. But my extra income was to help make the ends meet, not pay the mortgage. Overnight that all changed.

It was almost eerie. During our anniversary weekend, Mark and I were praying for a way for him to someday come home and join me. *But God . . . that wasn't what we had in mind!* He never went back to work again after that weekend.

We had a little money saved. It would keep us going for a few months, but then what? The answer came through the encouragement of a good friend in the packaging business, who pushed us to develop and market our own line of low-calorie, low-fat, high-fiber bagels. After prayerful consideration, Mark and I invested our meager savings to launch Kim's Light Foods and its flagship product, Kim's Light Bagels.

Had we known then what we know now, I don't think we would have *ever* had the guts to go through with it. Life got pretty scary for a while. Money was running out and winter weather was upon us. We couldn't afford an oil tank fill up, but learned that diesel fuel from the gas station was the same as home heating oil. My heart broke every time Mark took our five-gallon gas can up to the local gas station, filled it with diesel fuel, and poured it into the tank to keep the house warm for a few more days. The bagel launch was nearing, but would anyone buy them?

I remember saying to Mark, "You know, if these bagels don't sell we'll have 100,000 doggie-poop pick-up bags with my face on them!"

Thankfully, everyone else liked them as much as we did. Six months after our launch, Kim's Light Bagels were on nearly 1,000 grocery store shelves throughout the Northeast. We fulfill weekly online orders and have shipped bagels to all fifty states. The revenue from Kim's Light Bagels supports not only our household, but several others as well.

my story

The bagels brought more people to our Web site seeking weight loss motivation and encouragement. At last, we had the resources to launch our dream—online weight-loss meetings. Not just prerecorded programs, but LIVE meetings where people could chat together in real-time or call in and talk with me on air. I wanted to give them immediate feedback on their frustrations and cheer with them as they lost weight. I had seen how close online friendships could become, and I knew it would work if we could figure out how to do it.

"LIVE! With Kim" debuted its first weight-loss meeting on June 16, 2009. Right off the bat we had more than 500 people sign up, and more are joining us every day. Our offerings have grown to include other helpful tools like daily meal plans, shopping lists, recipes, and motivational video chats. Members were losing weight and staying on track when they had at other times fallen off.

I never thought all this would happen, and sometimes I can't believe it has. The rewards I've experienced through this freedom from food has made even more clear just how damaging the addiction is, and how much it steals from our lives. Of course, life still has its ups and downs, its highs and lows. They just aren't weight-related any more.

You can struggle with your weight for a lifetime, having tried "bajillions" of diets, surgeries or pills, shakes, and fasts. You can be a postmenopausal woman with hundreds of pounds to lose or an individual who hates exercise. It doesn't matter. You can still get to a healthy weight and stay there for the rest of your life. I wrote *Finally Thin!* because I want you to know that so badly, that I'm risking it all to tell you. Yes YOU! Believe. Find your hope. Try again. I know that it's not easy, but look at it this way:

DIETING IS HARD
BEING FAT IS HARD.
CHOOSE YOUR HARD.

This next section can help. Some of it you may have heard before, but it's worth repeating. Some of it may be completely new. Take from it what *you* need most on *your* journey to become finally thin because IT'S YOUR TURN NOW!

the **10** steps to a finally thin life

weight loss 101

I remember back in high school feeling fat all the time. I couldn't stop thinking about how much weight I had to lose and about how much larger I was than all of my friends. Today, I look back at photos taken during those years and I wonder what I was thinking. What was I looking at or comparing myself to? I looked normal. Not skinny, but certainly not overweight.

Does this sound familiar to you? I bet I'm not alone in this. Why was I so out of touch with how I really looked?

For many of us, though, the opposite is also true. Have you ever gone to a party or family gathering thinking that you looked pretty good—and been horrified later, when you saw a photograph of yourself, especially one taken from the back or the side or sitting down? And we think, "Holy cow. Literally . . . *holy cow!*"

Those are "final straw" moments—times when you come face to face with a harsh truth. Suddenly, you realize the only mirror you've been checking regularly is the one on your medicine chest—and it hasn't been telling you the whole story. For many of us, those photos showing the actual expanse of our girths come as a complete surprise. Moments like those, photos like those, send people racing to sign up for weight loss programs across America.

According to the latest statistics, 60 percent of all Americans are overweight (having a Body Mass Index of 25–29.9)—and 30 percent are obese (having a BMI of 30 or more). Those numbers are climbing rapidly, even as we spend billions of dollars on weight loss each year.

The fact that you're holding this book means that you are part of this giant industry. (I've dropped my fair share of disposable income into it, too.) It also probably means that you're still searching for answers. The best place to start is with a better understanding of how your body works. A tremendous amount of information is available, so let me help you sift through the key factors.

As a "professional dieter" I've waded through bajillions of handouts, pored over "Week One" books, tried to decipher "Phase Two" chapters, and downloaded endless pages online. If I only could have gotten credit for all that reading and those lectures—I'd certainly have a medical degree by now!

The best perspective I have to offer you as you get started is neutrality. I'm not here to sell you any one food plan or a particular weight loss program. I won't suggest one style or theory. I don't believe diets are one-size-fits-all. There are a lot of them on the market, and they all vary in amount of information, support, basic style, and theory. In my Diet Shoppe (page 67) you'll be able to see more clearly what they offer—and don't offer. It's a great place to go window shopping.

But first I want to focus on what you can expect from your body as you lose. Knowing these weight-loss basics will help you choose the best route for you—and keep you moving smoothly toward your destination.

weight loss by the numbers

For years, the standard way to know whether your weight was at a healthy number was to get on a scale and check your weight against a chart provided by the government. You ran your finger down the page to find your height and then moved it across to see what the normal weight range was for that height.

But even those charts were confusing. Years ago, some even asked women to measure themselves wearing two-inch heels (can you believe it?), and most had separate columns for small, medium, and large frames—but they didn't explain what that meant or how to figure it out.

Even Garfield, the cartoon cat, had an opinion on the subject when he said, "I'm not overweight, I'm undertall."

Today, although the height-weight range charts are still widely used, the medical community has gravitated toward another standard when determining healthy weights—the *body mass index,* or *BMI.*

The BMI is today's standard medical method of assessing healthy weight, overweight, and obesity. Although it is not always accurate for everyone (especially those with a high muscle mass or those under five feet tall), it is a quick and easy method for determining body fatness. To calculate your BMI, use the following formula:

$$BMI = \frac{\text{(weight in pounds)}}{\text{(height in inches)}^2} \times 703$$

(Note: This calculation is for adults only. Children and teens use a different formula that takes age and gender into consideration.)

height / weight / bmi chart

BMI	18.9 or Lower	19.0–24.9	25.0–29.9	30 or Higher
	Underweight	Healthy	Overweight	Obese
Height (in.)	Body Weight (lb.)			
	Less Than			More Than
58	90	91–118	119–142	143
59	93	94–123	124–147	148
60	96	97–127	128–152	153
61	99	100–131	132–157	158
62	103	104–135	136–163	164
63	106	107–140	141–168	169
64	109	110–144	145–173	174
65	113	114–149	150–179	180
66	117	118–154	155–185	186
67	120	121–157	158–190	191
68	124	125–163	164–197	198
69	127	128–168	169–202	203
70	131	132–173	174–208	209
71	135	136–178	179–214	215
72	139	140–183	184–220	221
73	143	144–188	189–226	227
74	147	148–193	194–232	233
75	151	152–199	200–239	240
76	155	156–204	205–245	246

SOURCE: www.nhlbi.nih.gov

the ten steps to a finally thin life

Weight = 140 lbs. Height = 5'5"

$[140 \div 65^2] \times 703 = 23.30$

This person has a BMI of 23.3, which reflects a healthy weight.

---

interpreting your BMI

- If your BMI is <19, you are **underweight.**

- If your BMI is 19 to 24.9, you have a **healthy weight.**

- If your BMI is 25 to 29.9, you are **overweight.**

- If your BMI is 30+, you are considered **obese.**

What's the difference between *overweight* and *obese?* If you check with a number of health organizations, you'll get a range of answers. Typically, if you are at least 20 percent over a healthy weight, you're considered obese (though some adjust it to say 25 percent for women). Now, most sources use the BMI of more than 30 to assess someone as obese.

Let's look at Susan's numbers. She knows she is overweight but is uncertain by how much.

EXAMPLE:

Weight = 210 lbs. Height = 5'6"

$[210 \div 66^2] \times 703 = 33.89$

Susan has a BMI of 33.89 and so is considered obese.

Susan needs to reduce her weight, but like most of us, she feels confused by the many diet programs available. Whom should she listen to? What is healthy? What will work for *her?*

Most of her options fall into two "camps"—the low-calorie programs and the low-carbohydrate plans. (Both of these generally encourage a reduction in the amount of fat consumed, though they permit varying amounts.)

finally thin!

No hard work equals no hard body.

camp one:
weight loss through calorie reduction

Many popular diets, such as Weight Watchers and Jenny Craig, are based on calorie reduction (even though you may not actually count calories). Because calorie counting seems like a lot of work, these programs provide plans that limit or eliminate the need to do it. What exactly is calorie counting?

A CALORIE IS A UNIT OF ENERGY. When it is related to food, a calorie (technically, a *kilocalorie)* measures the energy produced by food when it is *oxidized,* or burned as fuel by the body. When you take in more fuel than your body burns, the excess is stored in your body as fat. (And contrary to many misconceptions, a calorie is a calorie whether it comes from protein, fat, or carbohydrates.) To maintain weight you need to balance the energy you eat with the energy you use. Weight loss (or gain) is the result of an imbalance between calories in and calories out.

ONE POUND OF FAT EQUALS 3,500 CALORIES. In order to lose one pound of fat, you have to expend 3,500 more calories—or take in 3,500 fewer calories—than your body needs whether through increased activity, decreased eating, or both.

That's Weight Loss 101, according to the low-calorie camp.

If you know how many calories your body needs to maintain its current weight and you reduce that number by 500 calories each day, over a period of seven days you will lose one pound. If, in addition, you *burn* 500 calories each day through exercise, you will lose two pounds in a week.

You get the idea. It's simple math. Calorie counting is a form of dieting that has been around for years and is the "hidden science" behind many weight loss programs. They generally offer a "substitute" version of counting calories—points or exchanges, meal plans or units. But whatever they call it, it's generally based on the balance of calories in your body.

So how many calories does your body need? To determine that, we need to apply a formula to figure out your *basal metabolic rate,* or *BMR.*

basal metabolic rate (bmr)

Your basal metabolic rate (BMR) is an estimate of how many calories your body burns at rest. This represents the minimum number of calories your body needs on a daily basis to perform its most basic functions:

keeping your heart beating, regulating your breathing, and maintaining your body temperature. These are the calories burned just by being alive, and they account for 60 percent of the calories burned for an average person.

Although there are different formulas for calculating your BMR, the Mifflin–St. Jeor formula is considered the most accurate. It's not difficult, just a matter of plugging your numbers into the appropriate spots. (For those of you with math anxiety or no access to a calculator, you can *use the BMR calculator found on my site, www.kimbensen.com*)

Male:

(10 × weight in kilograms) + (6.25 × height in centimeters) –
(5 × age in years) + 5 =

Female:

(10 × weight in kilograms) + (6.25 × height in centimeters) –
(5 × age in years) – 161 =

EXAMPLE:

Female   Weight = 210 lbs. (95.25 kg)   Height = 5'5" (165.1 cm)   Age = 37

(10 × 95.25) + (6.25 × 165.1) – (5 × 37) – 161 = 1,639

= (952.5) + (1,031.9) – (185) – 161 = 1,639

= 1,639

Susan has a BMR of 1,638

conversions

1 pound = 0.45359237 kilograms (example: 210 lbs. × 0.45359237 = 95.25 kg)

1 foot = 2.54 centimeters (example: 65 in. × 2.54 = 165.1 cm)

Note: Your current BMR will go down as your age goes up or if your weight goes down. This means that as you get older or lose weight, your BMR will decrease and you will need to eat less and/or exercise more to maintain your current weight. Bummer.

finally thin!

As you are losing weight, you may want to refigure your BMR regularly. The BMR isn't the whole story. Your BMR represents the calories burned while at rest, but because very few people lie in bed all day, the next calculation will take activity level into consideration. To determine your total daily calorie needs, the BMR has to be multiplied by the appropriate activity factor. This number evaluates two things: energy expended during physical activity and the *thermogenetic effect* of food.

What does *thermogenetic effect* mean? Simply that 10 percent of your daily calories burned are burned in the process of eating, digesting, and utilizing food. *Yes,* you burn calories just by eating! I like to think of it as a 10 percent off sale at your favorite store. If you eat an apple for 70 calories, you expend 7 calories by biting, chewing, digesting, and using that apple for fuel for your body.

Now for the energy expended during physical activity. Use the following numbers to figure the actual number of calories you need to maintain your current weight. From there you can figure what you need to *lose* weight.

- If you are sedentary (little or no exercise): BMR × 1.2

- If you are lightly active (light exercise/sports 1–3 days/week): BMR × 1.375

- If you are moderately active (moderate exercise/sports 3–5 days/week): BMR × 1.55

- If you are very active (hard exercise/sports 6–7 days a week): BMR × 1.725

- If you are extra active (very hard exercise/sports, training): BMR × 1.9

EXAMPLE:

If Susan is moderately active, she will multiply her BMR × 1.55.

1,638 × 1.55 = 2,539

Her total number of daily calories needed to maintain her current weight is 2,539.

Note: This number is an estimate only. If you take certain medications, have excessive muscle mass, or deal with other health issues or genetic factors, the number produced by this calculation may not be completely accurate. Remember that weight loss is a very individual thing, and you may burn more or fewer calories than someone else while doing the same things. For most people, these calculations are an excellent starting point.

Many Web sites will calculate your BMI and BMR as well as the calories burned for various activities. My site, www.kimbensen.com, offers BMI and BMR calculators for those who don't want to do the math themselves or who want to double-check their numbers. Go ahead, it only takes a minute!

but what if you want to *lose* weight?

Your total daily calorie requirement is a great number to know if you want to maintain your current weight, but what if you want to lose weight? Now we come to *calorie reduction.* Once you've calculated your daily calorie needs, you can figure out how many calories to reduce in your diet, or burn in exercise!

Because you know that 3,500 calories equals a pound, you just need to determine how many calories you're willing to cut back on each day and/or how many calories you're willing to burn in exercise each day to achieve the results you want.

Begin by subtracting 20 percent of your daily calories. If Susan wants to lose weight, she can start by decreasing her daily calorie needs by 20 percent, or 0.2.

$$2,539 \times 0.2 = 508 \text{ calories}$$

That's 432 fewer calories each day or just under 3,500 calories in a week. We know that 3,500 calories equals one pound, so it should take Susan a bit more than one week to lose one pound.

However, if she also decides to *add* 500 calories' worth of exercise (calories burned) into her daily routine, the difference in her daily needs and what she is actually getting is close to 1,000 calories a day. That's nearly 7,000 calories, or two pounds, in a week. By reducing calories and adding exercise, Susan can double her potential weight loss results.

Most health professionals agree that 8 calories per pound of body weight is the rock bottom number, the fewest calories you should eat each day. Anything below that may compromise your health. A 135-lb. person would not want to go below 1,080 calories each day. Susan would not want to consume fewer than 1,680 calories.

Counting calories—and then reducing them—is a popular approach to weight loss. But plenty of research suggests that reducing carbohydrates is the key to lasting weight loss. Let's examine what these low-carb programs do.

camp two:
weight loss through carbohydrate reduction

Rather than cutting calories, low-carb diets such as Atkins, South Beach, and the Zone focus on reducing the amount of carbohydrates in your diet, replacing them with protein, fats, and fiber. On an annual basis, more than 26 million Americans spend more than $30 billion on low-carb products (*Time* magazine, "The Low-carb Food Craze," May 3, 2004). The basic premise behind the low-carb diet is that too many carbs can cause weight gain and discourage weight loss. Here are some of the reasons you may want to consider a low-carb program. (Besides the fact that carbs taste so darn good that they are hard to stop eating.)

how carbohydrates are metabolized by the body

Carbohydrates are one of the three main classifications of food (protein and fat are the other two) and a source of energy for the body. Carbohydrates are derived from the fiber, sugars, and starches found in foods such as bread, fruits, vegetables, dairy products, popcorn, potatoes, cookies, cake, and pasta.

During digestion, carbs are *metabolized* by the body—broken down to their simplest form, glucose, which is used by all cells, particularly brain cells, as fuel. When you eat simple carbs, your level of glucose rises quickly; when you eat complex carbs, this process happens more slowly, over a longer period of time—one of the reasons marathon runners are encouraged to eat pasta before a long race. Unfortunately, all carbs—good and bad—often get lumped together and are given a bad rap.

Once carbs are broken down to blood glucose, the pancreas automatically produces the hormone insulin. This causes the liver to convert the glucose into glycogen and triglycerides, whose job it is to bring your blood sugar back to normal levels. Your body stores glucose reserves in the muscles in the form of glycogen, ready to be used when you exert yourself. Unless you are diabetic, you're unlikely to give this process a second thought.

reducing carbohydrate intake

Because one function of the hormone insulin is to help the body store glucose as fat, lowering your carbohydrate consumption will result in the pancreas secreting less insulin and thus storing less fat. When carbs are restricted, glucose levels do not rise. Instead of producing more insulin, the pancreas increases production of the hormone glucagon. Glucagon uses the glycogen and triglycerides (stored fat reserves) in the body as a new energy source or fuel. The liver begins to break down the extra fatty acids, producing energy for the body in the form of ketones and glucose. Being in *ketosis* means that your body's primary source of energy is fat in the form of ketones. Ketosis means high levels of these ketones in the blood.

> Counting carbs is easy using the food label. Just take the total carbohydrate grams and subtract the fiber and sugar alcohol grams. The remaining carb grams are the product's "net carbs."

There are benefits to low-carb living other than weight loss. The presence of ketones in the bloodstream often results in decreased appetite. (Who doesn't want *that?*) *And* low-carb diets are often higher in fat. Fat takes the body longer to digest than carbs and gives you a feeling of fullness for a longer time. And let's not forget how good fat makes food taste!

However, experts caution that there may also be side effects when the body is in a state of ketosis. These can include headaches, increased urination, constipation and dehydration, more rapid fatigue during exercise, and bad breath. Long-term concerns may include increased bone loss, according to a 2007 study.

Recent research questions how low you need to go when eating low carb. Some low-carb diets deliver similar results while producing different levels of ketosis. The Atkins program, for instance, can be a very low-carbohydrate diet—less than 20 grams of net carbs daily—and is ketogenic (produces ketosis), while the Zone diet, promoting a more moderate intake of carbs (up to 180 grams of net carbs) is nonketogenic and may provide dieters with increased energy that provides greater stamina during fitness activities.

the glycemic index (gi) in brief

Some carbohydrates raise your blood sugar level quickly (that's *bad*), while others take longer to break down and raise it only slightly (that's *good*). In 1981, Dr. David J. Jenkins and colleagues at the University of Toronto developed the *glycemic index (GI)*, which ranks carbohydrates according to their effect on blood glucose in the first hours after consumption.

The GI compares carbohydrates gram for gram in individual foods and provides a numerical value calculated from data collected from a small number of subjects whose blood was taken and evaluated after a meal. The result was a relative ranking for each tested food.

Foods with low-GI ratings, such as most vegetables, beans, and whole grains that have a higher fiber content, make your blood glucose rise and fall gently; eating them can reduce your appetite and cravings. High-GI foods, including white bread, white potatoes, and cake, whose carbs have been highly refined and processed, are broken down quickly by the body; these foods cause blood glucose levels to surge and then crash, leaving you feeling unsatisfied after a short amount of time.

eating for good health versus eating for weight loss

Healthy eating means different things to different people and can be done on many levels. For some, healthy eating means staying within your calorie range and consuming an assortment of vitamins, minerals, and nutrients from all the food groups in proportion to what the body needs. You lose weight—get healthier—by healthy eating.

To others it's all about a lack of processed foods and additives and selecting from choice, organic products.

Eating "healthy" and eating for weight loss are not necessarily the same thing. They *can* be, but they aren't always. Many people think of healthy eating as selecting organic foods and whole grains and would turn their noses up at anything with processed carbs or refined sugars. My concern when I was losing weight was not health food as much as weight loss, pure and simple. What I loved about my diet was that I *could* eat *some* nachos or birthday cake or whatever processed carbs I wanted, if I so chose. Today, although counting calories is still the number one factor in how I choose what I eat, I am also starting to look more closely at the ingredients in the foods I select.

Here is a word of advice, however. Even you low-calorie lovers should limit your processed carbs. Eating 1,200 calories a day may give you the weight loss you desire, but if you're eating 70 percent carbohydrates, 10 percent fats, and 20 percent everything else, you're not eating healthy.

It also makes sense for low-carb lovers to be cautious with fats. Even if you are "permitted" to eat a huge steak wrapped in bacon, you may want to be selective about how often you indulge in that particular delight. Digesting all that fat can be hard on your body!

Simply put, whether you choose to live low calorie, low fat, low carb, or a combination of the three, it is still important to eat for good health, not simply for weight loss. That's why I think choosing from a wide variety of healthy food plans is so important. We are all different. Go all-organic. Go low carb. Go low calorie. But *go!*

exercise is a weight loss basic

"How much did you exercise?" I get asked this question all the time.

The good news is: I didn't exercise.

The bad news is: I didn't exercise. At least not much.

I say this because although it is possible to lose weight without exercise (yeah!), exercise offers many benefits far beyond weight loss. Exercise will help you tone the outside of the body you are reshaping with weight loss—and it can make a real difference to the enduring health of what's inside: your heart, your muscles, your lungs, and even your brain!

Another benefit of exercise is that you can "earn" the opportunity to eat more. That's an important plus when it comes to working toward long-term weight loss and maintenance. Remember, as you lose weight, you need fewer calories to maintain your body, but increasing your physical activity makes greater demands for fuel—and so you can *add* calories to your daily menu.

Here's another reason to exercise: It increases the body's BMR. As you build muscle, you burn more calories, and you continue to burn more calories after you finish exercising. Your BMR is directly linked to the amount of muscle your body has. The more muscle you have, the higher your BMR. In other words, any exercise you perform has benefits that last far beyond the actual calories you burn doing it.

So not only do you reap the benefits from every activity through the actual calories you burn as you go, you also increase your body's muscle tone. This goes for cardiovascular activity, which builds muscle tone in your heart, and for strength training, which builds muscle tone in your abs, your arms, your legs, your back—all over. It's *all* muscle.

You may love to exercise. You feel invigorated and alive when you start your day out with a brisk walk, or you can't wait to hit the gym at lunch. That's wonderful, and there are so many of us who *envy* you! Keep up the great work. If you've never been able to join the "love to exercise" club no matter how many programs you've tried or tapes you've purchased, don't despair. By starting with small commitments you, too, can make exercise part of your healthier new life. That's exactly what I did.

Okay. You've finished Weight Loss 101. Are you ready to start your journey to a healthy weight and better health? Let's look at some of the options out there and choose a diet that's a great fit for you.

1

choose the diet
that's right for you

Some people will tell you, "Never say diet!" Guess what. Everyone diets. If you look up the term *diet* in the dictionary, the first definition is "food and drink regularly provided or consumed." So whether you're getting guidance through a formal program with the goal of reducing your weight or choosing what you eat simply based on desire, that is your diet. Diet is *not* a four-letter word. Well, it is, but you know what I mean.

If you are able to cut back on your portions and eliminate certain foods in a balanced way on your own to lose weight, that's wonderful. Most of us need a little more structure than that. If we didn't, we wouldn't be still struggling with our weight. That's where choosing a diet program comes in.

choosing a weight loss plan
that's right for you

So where do we start? There are just *so many* different diets out there—how can you be sure that the one you choose is the right one for you?

Let's start with some questions about who you are and how you feel about weight loss. I'm confident that if you've bought this book, you've struggled with one or more of the major weight loss issues: proper daily nutrition, portion sizes, healthy activity levels, and behavioral issues that seem to affect anyone on a diet.

Many say if you "just" cut back on your intake and increase your output, you will lose weight. No diet needed. True? True! However, I have to be honest: If I could have done that, I would have a long time ago. For those of us who have trouble recognizing physical fullness (or trouble stopping when we know we're full), the framework and guidelines a diet offers are a necessity. If you've been trying to lose weight and haven't yet succeeded in losing the weight you want and keeping it off, finding a good diet plan is a great place to start.

Whether you go low calorie or low carbohydrate, vegetarian or all meat, you will lose weight over time because you are cutting your intake in one form or another. But dieting and dieting *healthfully* are definitely not the same thing.

A lot of very good diets are available, but mixed in with those are plenty of unhealthy ones. I know. I've tried most of them.

Here are three things *everyone* should consider when selecting a diet plan:

1. is it healthy?

DOES IT INCORPORATE ALL THE FOOD GROUPS AND PROVIDE ENOUGH CALORIES FOR YOUR AGE, WEIGHT, AND ACTIVITY LEVEL? Most medical experts recommend a minimum of 1,200 calories daily. Diets eliminating entire food groups typically end up eliminating vital minerals, protein, and vitamins. Diets based on only one food, such as grapefruit or cabbage, are not only boring but also nutritionally lacking. They tend to be fad diets that should be avoided. A wide variety of foods ensures that you receive the nutrients you need.

How to spot a fad diet:

Eliminates entire food groups

Lacks variety

Foods claim to "burn fat"

Foods promise to increase metabolism

Diets with increased caffeine intake

Promises a fast or unrealistic weight loss

Does not suggest consulting your doctor

Does not recommend increased activity or lifestyle changes

IS EXERCISE PART OF THE PLAN? If the diet plan you choose does not include a recommendation for exercise, make sure you plan at some point to include it as part of your overall healthy lifestyle. The boost that exercise gives your metabolism is helpful in long-term weight control. You can lose without it, but you'll probably lose more slowly, and you'll be less likely to keep the weight off. But there are far more benefits to exercise than just weight loss, and a healthy daily routine is something we should all strive for.

HOW MUCH WEIGHT CAN YOU EXPECT TO LOSE PER WEEK? This is a very individual thing. Much depends on who you are, how active you are, how faithful you are to the diet, and how much you weigh. Beware of diets that promise speedy, effortless weight loss, without exercise and/or without changes in your eating behavior. Experts advise that

choosing your diet—a lifestyle quiz

Which diet is best for you? Take the quiz and find out!
Think through what's important to you as you answer the questions in the following quiz. The results will help point you in the right direction, or at least help you narrow your choices.

Next, head to the Diet Shoppe (page 67) and see which of the programs listed best match your needs and desires. Think of it as weight-loss matchmaking.

What do you want in a diet? Check all the ones that apply:
- ☐ Low-calorie food plan
- ☐ Low-carb food plan
- ☐ Packaged food
- ☐ A program that tells me exactly what and when to eat
- ☐ A program that lets me pick and choose my own food
- ☐ A program with an emphasis on cooking
- ☐ Help with behavioral modification
- ☐ Education about good nutrition
- ☐ Strong exercise emphasis
- ☐ Easy to follow
- ☐ Low cost

losing weight too fast can be hard on the body and ultimately un-healthy. As wonderful as it would be to lose weight quickly, the facts are clear: weight lost in a slow, steady way is healthier and more likely to be sustained.

ARE SUPPLEMENTS INVOLVED? Any diet based on pills, shakes, or sup-plements rarely offers more than a temporary weight loss fix. Are you prepared to purchase and consume those products for the rest of your life? If not, as soon as you stop taking them, the weight loss is likely to stop as well. And you should always run these types of weight loss plans past your health care provider before taking them.

WHAT DOES YOUR DOCTOR RECOMMEND? Do you have specific medical needs that would be better adapted to one diet program over an-

What support/tools would best help you?

☐ Group or individual meetings
☐ Physician supervision
☐ Online support
☐ Planning/tracking tools
☐ Specific exercise routines/schedule
☐ Recipes
☐ Meal planning
☐ Grocery shopping ideas and lists
☐ A program with a spiritual emphasis

How would you best describe your preferred eating habits?

☐ Grazing throughout the day, including several small meals
☐ Three meals plus snacks
☐ Heavy nighttime eating
☐ Eating on the run
☐ Eating out more than three times a week
☐ Organic/natural ingredients

the ten steps to a finally thin life

other? Ask your health care provider for suggestions about specific diets that have been shown to produce the results you want (for example, someone with cardiac concerns may be encouraged to choose a diet designed for that purpose).

2. do you *like* it?

ASK YOURSELF, "IS THIS SOMETHING I CAN DO AND LIVE WITH FOR THE REST OF MY LIFE?" If the answer is no, then it's probably not the plan for you. Diets provide a wonderful structure that many of us lack in our daily eating regimens—part of the reason we are overweight in the first place. But unless the structure of a particular diet can be woven into the fabric of your life and become an integral part of who you are and how you eat, it will never become that new and enduring lifestyle you are seeking. *Enjoyment* is the gateway to a healthy lifestyle that *lasts.*

IS COUNTING INVOLVED—POINTS OR CALORIES OR CARBS? Keeping track of what you eat, all day, every day, takes commitment. Will you do it? If not, move on.

WILL YOU BE REQUIRED TO EAT ANY FOOD ITEMS THAT YOU JUST CAN'T STOMACH? A diet that includes two meals a day of a particular shake or bar won't work for you unless you find it tasty and satisfying.

3. is it a good fit?

DOES IT FIT YOUR PERSONALITY, YOUR NEEDS, YOUR LIFE? There are many healthy and enjoyable programs, but they're *not* all right for you. If you don't have the time or interest to do major food preparation or planning, programs like NutriSystem or Zone Chef might be a good fit. But if you're a single mom working two jobs to make ends meet, a prepared food delivery program is unlikely to fit into your budget. You might love the idea of meals arriving on your doorstep, but if you can't afford it, the financial stress may drive you to the cookie jar!

WHAT ABOUT SUPPORT? Any program you choose should help you set realistic goals and offer you information on behavior modification to help get you there. We all need some kind of support, but think about what kind will help you the most. Do you need the accountability of stepping on a scale each week and having your weight officially recorded? That worked for me, along with the rah-rah at my weekly meeting and the guidance of a leader, but everyone is different. Some affordable self-help support groups include Overeaters Anonymous and Take Off Pounds Sensibly (TOPS). You may get the support you need at a fraction of the cost of other programs.

ARE YOU SINGLE? COOKING FOR A CROWD? Some programs may be so strict about cooking methods that you'll need to prepare one meal for yourself and something else for family members whose nutritional needs differ from yours. Can you commit to doing all that extra work?

DO YOU COOK FOR SOMEONE WITH FOOD ALLERGIES OR WHO IS DIABETIC? ARE THERE OTHER DIETARY RESTRICTIONS IN THE HOUSEHOLD TO TAKE INTO CONSIDERATION? If you're already making special dishes for someone else, you may need a plan that fits in with what you are doing, one that is utterly simple, or one that uses frozen or packaged foods to supplement what you are already doing.

HOW WILL YOUR WORK ENVIRONMENT, YOUR SCHEDULE, AND YOUR SOCIAL LIFE MESH WITH A PARTICULAR DIET? If you need to entertain clients frequently or travel often, that may influence your choice of food plan.

diet shoppe

Fad diets come and go faster than you can say "water weight." With so many "new," "improved," and "revolutionary" diets popping up on the market each year, it's no wonder that people feel confused. My Diet Shoppe is a comprehensive tool designed to help you sort through the possibilities. With just a quick glance, you'll learn the basic facts about more than twenty-five popular diets available to you. Kind of like window shopping! *There is something here for everyone.*

Here's a peek at all the diets out there. Browse. Then choose what works for you!

the 3-hour diet

THE SKINNY: Originated by Jorge Cruise, this diet is designed so that you eat every three hours, which is supposed to improve metabolism and promote greater loss of fat. The goal is to have your body burn fat instead of muscle as fuel. The plan emphasizes portion control and planning ahead to eat well-balanced meals and snacks. You don't have to count carbs or fat grams. All foods are permitted, so you can choose what you want to combat cravings.

WHAT'S GOOD: Cruise provides several different approaches, depending on your interests and needs: a heart-healthy version, and a version for people who want or need to eat fast foods.

WHAT'S NOT SO GOOD: For people who aren't careful about portion control, it can be easy to overdo. Cruise recommends his exercise program, 8-Minute Moves, but some experts feel it's too short to provide needed calorie burning.

THE COST: The cost of the book plus groceries.

the abs diet

THE SKINNY: From the editor of *Men's Health* magazine, this is a six-meals-per-day program that suggests you'll lose belly fat first. The diet uses an acronym to remind you what to eat:

Almonds and other nuts
Beans and other legumes
Spinach and other green veggies

Dairy (fat free or low fat)
Instant unsweetened oatmeal
Eggs
Turkey and other lean meat

Peanut butter
Olive oil
Whole-grain bread and cereal
Extra protein from whey powder
Raspberries and other berries

The author recommends you consume whey protein powder along with these "power foods" and do thirty minutes of exercise several times a week, including weight training and some cardio.

WHAT'S GOOD: The author recommends a fairly complete program of healthy eating and exercise laid out in a simple, flexible way. Both the interactive Web site and the book have easy-to-follow illustrations of the author's recommended exercises.

WHAT'S NOT SO GOOD: The Web site claims "turn fat into muscle," which is not physically possible as they are two separate things. It also claims you will lose from your stomach first, which, is also impossible as there is no such thing as specific spot reduction— unfortunately.

THE COST: The cost of the book plus groceries. The online component has a thirty-day free trial, but unless you sign up there is no indication of the ongoing costs.

the atkins diet

THE SKINNY: On the Atkins diet, you'll eat as much protein as you want, including meats, eggs, and cheese, as well as fats, including mayonnaise, butter, and oils. You'll have to limit carbohydrates to a bare minimum, including pasta, potatoes, bread, and fruit. There are four stages to the Atkins diet: Induction, Ongoing Weight Loss, Pre-Maintenance, and Lifetime Maintenance. Each stage becomes progressively less restrictive and gradually increases carbohydrates allowed.

WHAT'S GOOD: Weight loss can be fast, especially at the start. You'll enjoy foods that are often restricted from diets such as bacon and real sour cream. You may feel satisfied longer because you're eating high-fat foods. It's basically easy to follow. Online support is available. Dining out is easy (though *not* eating the rolls can be challenging).

WHAT'S NOT SO GOOD: Many foods are eliminated, including bread, rice, and alcohol. The saturated fat in meat can be bad for your heart. Your breath may smell of the ketones being released by your body. Some dieters have reported feeling low in energy; others complained of hair loss and fast weight gain when they went off the diet. Some have noted constipation (because you're eating low fiber). Most people who follow Atkins end up eating very high fat, promoting concerns from the medical community about cardiac health.

THE COST: The cost of the book plus groceries. It can be expensive to consume so much protein.

the best life diet (bob greene)

THE SKINNY: This is the program designed by Oprah's fitness trainer. He divides the diet into three phases:

First phase: He has you make gradual changes in your lifestyle, including eating three meals and one snack daily. He insists that you eat breakfast, increase activity, skip alcohol, take vitamins, and stop eating two hours before you go to bed.

Second phase: Now you're on a true weight loss diet, eliminating unhealthy foods, planning menus, working out more.

Third phase: This is when you make your commitment for life.

WHAT'S GOOD: You keep a journal of what you eat and how you feel. If you join the Web site, you have access to all kinds of support, including recipes and a message board. Bob Greene is a good motivator, and if you "get with the program" and stay with it, you should lose and keep the weight off.

WHAT'S NOT SO GOOD: Some critics noted that Bob recommends some branded food items, but you don't have to use them.

THE COST: The cost of the book and your groceries plus approximately $4.50 per week to use the Web site.

the blood type diet (eat right for your blood type)

THE SKINNY: This diet says that your blood type can influence how you lose weight and that you should emphasize certain foods if you want to be successful. The diet lists very specific foods you should and should not eat. For example, those with blood type A should go vegetarian while type O should eliminate grains. You're also told to exercise based on your blood type, more than by what you enjoy.

WHAT'S GOOD: Some users report renewed energy.

WHAT'S NOT SO GOOD: Critics believe there is no valid scientific proof behind this program. You have to eliminate many healthy foods depending on which blood type you are and could miss out on needed nutrients. It can be very difficult for members of the same family to eat the same foods if their blood types differ.

THE COST: The price of the book plus the cost of preparing different meals for your family.

the cabbage soup diet

THE SKINNY: This diet keeps coming around and, not surprisingly, no one group seems to want to claim responsibility. It consists of a vegetable soup that you consume in unlimited amounts for a week. The promise is that you'll lose ten to fifteen pounds during that week. The plan usually adds some other foods to the soup (potatoes, fruits, beef) on different days, but mostly it's just soup.

WHAT'S GOOD: Eating vegetables is good, and you will drop weight, primarily because you're reducing your calorie intake to the extreme.

WHAT'S NOT SO GOOD: Most people gain the weight back quickly. Many report feeling weak and dizzy during the seven days. Expect to spend a lot of time in the bathroom. Your body may suffer from a lack of nutrients if you use it long-term.

THE COST: Just the cost of food. You can print the recipe out from the Internet.

curves

THE SKINNY: This diet seeks to reset your set point* and was created by the founder of the Curves gyms. You'll need to exercise at least ninety minutes a week and follow a specific diet plan.

WHAT'S GOOD: The food plan is flexible and asks you to think about your food triggers. It provides shopping lists and recipes, and you'll eat six meals a day. Dieters are encouraged to keep a journal and set interim goals. If you join a Curves gym you will have the support of their staff and the community of fellow members.

*The set point theory claims that your body has a memory of a comfortable metabolism which can be reset at a higher level through managing what and when we eat, thereby making weight loss easier. This is a debated concept and its popularity seems to swing back and forth.

WHAT'S NOT SO GOOD: Curves products are marketed throughout the book, including shakes, vitamins, and other items. (You don't have to buy them.)

THE COST: The cost of the book and your groceries plus the optional costs of belonging to Curves and buying their products, if you choose. The online component is $5 per week.

dean ornish's eat more to weigh less

THE SKINNY: Dean Ornish is one of the top authorities on avoiding heart disease, so you can feel confident that his recommendations are research based. He prescribes exercise and vitamins plus supplements. The diet is strict: vegetarian, focusing on fruits, vegetables, grains, beans, and nonfat dairy—and no meat, no oil, no nuts, no alcohol.

WHAT'S GOOD: This is a high-fiber, low-fat diet. Ornish's patients have seen improvement in their cardiac status and have lost weight.

WHAT'S NOT SO GOOD: This is a difficult diet for most people to stick to because it eliminates many popular foods and is very restrictive. It's hard to eat out on this program, though some have managed it.

THE COST: Just the cost of the book plus groceries. If you have medical concerns, you may have to add the cost of tests to confirm that it's working for you.

dr. andrew weil's optimum health plan

THE SKINNY: This program from a Harvard Medical School professor focuses on holistic eating and draws from Eastern as well as Western health care. You eat a comprehensive meal plan including lean proteins, fruits, and vegetables and good carbs.

WHAT'S GOOD: The foods are healthy, the Web site offers lots of holistic support for dieters and nondieters, and the emphasis on non-processed foods is a strong one.

WHAT'S NOT SO GOOD: Dr. Weil does sell supplements, and not all dieters may want to deal with the constant "sell" on the Web site. He also recommends more calories per day than may produce the kind of weight loss many dieters seek.

THE COST: The cost of the book and groceries plus any supplements purchased. The online Web subscription plan is $4 per week with a four-week minimum.

dr. phil's ultimate weight solution

THE SKINNY: Subtitled the Seven Keys to Weight Loss Freedom, this book and plan came from the popular television host whose straight-forward, no-nonsense philosophy to life is the approach he takes in his weight loss advice. He emphasizes behavior management and tackles emotional eating. He encourages dieters to eat high-fiber foods— fruits, vegetables, grains—as well as lean proteins and healthy fats.

WHAT'S GOOD: The diet focuses on healthy food choices and can work well for eaters whose greatest challenge is emotional, not physical. He includes case studies and self-tests and encourages journaling to help change old habits.

WHAT'S NOT SO GOOD: Dr. Phil was criticized for promoting many weight loss products, including shakes, bars, and vitamins.

THE COST: The cost of the book and groceries plus optional purchases of recommended products.

exchange plans

THE SKINNY: This category includes early versions of Weight Watchers, Richard Simmons, many government programs, and diabetic eating plans. JoAnna Lund's Healthy Exchanges fits in here as well. Ex-change programs provide you with lists of foods in different cate-gories and tell you how many from each category you're allowed each day.

WHAT'S GOOD: Some dieters find this method easier to follow than many other diet plans. A number of diet tools help you keep track of how many exchanges you've eaten and how many you still have to go. Exchange plans also help dieters create menus that include all the food groups.

WHAT'S NOT SO GOOD: Some dieters get fed up with the constant counting. They may also get in a rut of eating the same foods week after week.

THE COST: The cost of groceries plus any books you choose to purchase. However, you can print most of these plans for free from the Internet.

the fat flush plan

THE SKINNY: This is a detox plan that evolves into a diet. During the first Two-Week Fat Flush phase, your goal through an 1,100-calorie-per-day diet is to lose bloat. The second Ongoing Fat Flush phase increases the calories to 1,500 per day. Finally, you learn how to eat for maintenance on the Lifestyle Eating Plan, where good carbs are introduced.

WHAT'S GOOD: The program pushes exercise and eight hours of sleep per night. The foods are healthy, if limited.

WHAT'S NOT SO GOOD: Not everyone loves consuming the psyllium "Long Life" cocktail that is part of the plan. The calorie counts are low, which can discourage people from sticking to the plan long-term.

THE COST: The cost of the book plus food and the psyllium supplements.

first place

THE SKINNY: First Place describes itself as a Christ-centered, balanced weight loss program that has guided hundreds of thousands of people to a healthy lifestyle and a closer walk with the Lord. Its Web site outlines a program that includes Bible study, group support, and accountability; a commonsense nutrition plan; regular exercise; daily prayer; and Scripture memorization. Members are asked to make "commitments" when joining a class:

- Attendance

- Encouragement

- Prayer

- Bible reading

- Scripture memory

- Bible study

- "Live-It" plan

- Commitment record

- Exercise

WHAT'S GOOD: The diet promotes low-fat, well-balanced eating and exercise. Dieters looking for a faith-based program will find this very comprehensive. Those who feel that their success in long-term weight loss is directly related to their faith may respond to this program when they've had difficulty sticking to other plans.

WHAT'S NOT SO GOOD: Groups may be led by anyone who is inclined to do so and who purchases a Group Starter Kit.

THE COST: Besides groceries, all members must invest in a one-time purchase of a Member's Kit ($79.99) that includes lots of support materials, including motivational CDs, plus a supplemental Bible study package ($19.99) every ten weeks.

food combining

THE SKINNY: These diets tell you not to eat carbs with proteins, or recommend you eat fruit and then wait two hours to eat another kind of food. The Beverly Hills diet was a popular one of these; Suzanne Somers's program (discussed later) is another.

WHAT'S GOOD: People who prefer not to measure portions often like these programs, which let you choose the amount as long as you don't mix what shouldn't be mixed. Also, you will be eating lots of fruits and vegetables.

WHAT'S NOT SO GOOD: There isn't much research showing that food combining works better than other methods, though many dieters say they feel better when they don't mix. You need to be careful not to miss out on important nutrients.

THE COST: The cost of the book, if you choose to purchase a copy, plus groceries. You can also find the details online.

french women don't get fat

THE SKINNY: This recent bestseller is a way of eating that imitates what French women supposedly do to stay thin: eat smaller portions, eat in moderation, and exercise regularly.

WHAT'S GOOD: The program encourages portion control, and by not denying dieters foods they may crave (cheese, chocolate), the likelihood of bingeing is diminished. Eaters are also taught to enjoy food, eat slowly, eat fresh, and keep a journal. The online program offers daily meal plans, recipes, an interactive journal, and tips from author Mireille Guiliano.

WHAT'S NOT SO GOOD: It does not address emotional eating. The dieter must exercise lots of self-discipline in order to make this program work long-term.

THE COST: The cost of the book plus good-quality foods. The online membership costs $19.95 per month.

the grapefruit diet (aka mayo clinic diet)

THE SKINNY: This classic diet is essentially a low-calorie diet that suggests that eating half a grapefruit before each meal, drinking water, and eating a specific combination of foods will cause weight loss.

WHAT'S GOOD: You're getting lots of vitamin C with your daily citrus.

WHAT'S NOT SO GOOD: Grapefruit can interfere with many prescription drugs. Also, this diet is very low in calories, protein, and fiber. No diet should rely so heavily on one food. It is unclear whether the Grapefruit Diet and the original Mayo Clinic Diet are just similar or the same fad diet. Either way, neither is endorsed by the renowned Mayo Clinic and is not to be confused with the Mayo Clinic Plan, which is available in book form only.

THE COST: The diet is available for free on the Internet; the cost of grapefruit varies from season to season.

high-protein diets

THE SKINNY: These diets eliminate or severely limit carbohydrates. They appeal to dieters who crave meat and who resist eating fruits and vegetables. The theory is that when you reduce the carbs you consume, the body will burn fat for energy.

WHAT'S GOOD: Weight loss can be fast, and eating fat and protein can make restaurant eating easier.

WHAT'S NOT SO GOOD: Because you are eating little fiber, you may experience constipation. High-protein diets have been linked to increased cholesterol; the high saturated fat that often comes with them can have cardiac implications.

THE COST: Information can be found for free on the Internet; buying large quantities of protein can be expensive.

jenny craig

THE SKINNY: With celebrity spokespeople such as Sara Rue and Valerie Bertinelli, this diet program has gotten lots of recent attention. You eat frozen or shelf-stable packaged foods, supplemented with some fresh items. You meet with Jenny Craig staff for regular motivational sessions and weigh-ins.

WHAT'S GOOD: Ease of preparation; the meals are prepared for you, so no measuring or planning is required; weekly consultations are a source of support.

WHAT'S NOT SO GOOD: The counselors are not medical professionals; the commitment to eating packaged foods is pricey; you get little practice in preparing food yourself or learning to dine sensibly in restaurants; portion sizes can be small; and it can be expensive over time.

THE COST: The weekly commitment is only $5, but the food can cost from $75 each week to well over $100—and you still need to supplement with other groceries.

juice fasts

THE SKINNY: Used by some dieters as a short-term fix, juice fasts eliminate all solid foods and consist of fresh and bottled juices only. Although they provide more nutrition than a total fast, they are not to be used for the longer term.

WHAT'S GOOD: If you've been overeating lots of unhealthy foods, a two-day juice fast can be a cleansing launch to a healthier eating plan.

WHAT'S NOT SO GOOD: You will likely feel weak and dizzy and may experience headaches as you get rid of toxins. You'll also feel hunger pangs for at least the first day or so. It's difficult to eat out anywhere but a juice bar.

THE COST: If you own a juicer, you'll pay only for quantities of fruits and vegetables. If not, a good-quality juicer is more than $200. If you purchase all your juices, you may spend as much for them as you would for regular meals out.

low-fat diets

THE SKINNY: Many diets can be considered low in fat, even if that is not their focus. If you're concerned about heart health and want to lower your cholesterol, consider a diet program that specifically limits the amount of fat you take in.

WHAT'S GOOD: Low-fat diets tend to emphasize high-fiber foods that deliver more of a sense of fullness; high-fat foods, even if permitted, are allowed in such small quantities that they may not seem "worth it."

WHAT'S NOT SO GOOD: You need a certain amount of fat to keep your body healthy and prevent your skin and hair from being too dry. But you can get that amount of fat from lean proteins.

THE COST: Sometimes reduced-fat foods cost more than the regular kinds.

the mayo clinic plan

THE SKINNY: Not to be confused with the fad Mayo Clinic Diet. This program *is* endorsed by the Mayo Clinic and is based on their Healthy Weight Pyramid. It recommends eating foods with low energy density—those that contain a small number of calories in a large amount of food, such as fruits, vegetables, legumes, poultry, fish, and whole grains.

WHAT'S GOOD: Designed by medical professionals from a reputable health institute. They offer personalized menus, shopping lists, meal plans, results charts, and dining-out tips.

WHAT'S NOT SO GOOD: Excellent in diet and exercise, but could be stronger in behavior modification, motivation, and emotional support.

THE COST: Just the cost of the book plus groceries.

nutrisystem

THE SKINNY: The NutriSystem Nourish program uses the glycemic index to encourage dieters to enjoy good carbs and keep fat low. You order packaged foods and supplement them with fresh fruits and vegetables. Portion control is built in.

WHAT'S GOOD: You can get phone support from a dietitian. It's all about convenience. The meals are prepared for you so if you don't want to cook for yourself or if you are too busy, this solves that problem.

WHAT'S NOT SO GOOD: You get no practice living without the prepared foods, portion sizes can be small, and it can be expensive over time.

THE COST: The program costs approximately $289 for thirty days' worth of food. QVC sells a four-week package with weekends off for just over $180. It also features a one-week package of favorites for $76.

overeaters anonymous

THE SKINNY: This is a twelve-step program for people who identify themselves as powerless over food (including compulsive overeaters, anorexics, bulimics, and binge eaters).

WHAT'S GOOD: You take a questionnaire to evaluate your relationship with food. The program provides a set of tools for recovery, which include eating from an eating plan, meeting with a sponsor, reviewing the literature, giving service, and prayer. OA provides six different eating plans.

WHAT'S NOT SO GOOD: Not everyone is comfortable with the philosophy of OA that requires accepting powerlessness.

THE COST: Attendance at OA meetings is free. OA is supported by member contributions. The only cost is groceries.

perricone prescription

THE SKINNY: This monthlong program claims to improve your skin at the cellular level by changing to an anti-inflammatory, antioxidant-rich diet, which can help with risks of heart disease, arthritis, cancer, diabetes, and obesity. Foods that rank high on the glycemic index (potatoes, pasta, bread) are eliminated to prevent wrinkles and aging of skin.

WHAT'S GOOD: Dr. Perricone encourages dieters to eat three meals and two snacks each day and to get regular exercise.

WHAT'S NOT SO GOOD: The program is twenty-eight days long and requires that you eat salmon almost every day. It is heavy on supplementation, and Dr. Perricone's claims of "being wrinkle free for life" have been questioned by experts.

THE COST: The cost of the book plus the required foods (salmon is expensive!), also the cost of the supplements if you choose to use them.

picture perfect diet (dr. shapiro)

THE SKINNY: Dr. Shapiro's book focuses on making smart food choices, in part by using photos to compare servings of equivalent calorie value. He encourages dieters to eat for volume satisfaction with healthy, high-fiber foods. He also makes regular exercise a part of the equation and stresses that dieters need to get at the emotional reasons behind overeating in order to ensure long-term weight loss.

WHAT'S GOOD: This is a sensible, healthy approach to weight loss that can produce results because the picture-perfect photos have a tremendous impact.

WHAT'S NOT SO GOOD: The book discourages dairy products, recommending soy products instead, which may not be right for everyone.

It also suggests that you'll experience fast results, which is unlikely for most dieters.

THE COST: Just the cost of the book plus groceries.

prepared meals

THE SKINNY: This is not a diet plan but instead an eating option based on calorie-controlled packaged foods—primarily frozen entrées but potentially including a variety of packaged food products. It's fast food for weight loss.

WHAT'S GOOD: Packaged foods work as part of many popular diet programs, and they are widely available. They also offer tremendous variety. If you're incredibly busy and cooking only for yourself, they can be a real help. Fans of this kind of dieting highlight the quick preparation and easy cleanup.

WHAT'S NOT SO GOOD: Packaged foods tend to be high in sodium, so using them more than occasionally can really add up. Also, costs can be high and servings quite small and thus not satisfying. Eating them doesn't prepare you for cooking and eating away from the microwave.

THE COST: Most frozen entrées cost from $2.50 to $5.00 each. Supplementing these meals with other food items can increase your grocery bill.

the pritikin diet

THE SKINNY: Created by an expert in treating heart disease, the Pritikin program is a very low-fat, mostly vegetarian food plan that emphasizes fruits, vegetables, and whole grains. A later edition adds back healthy fats, which were not a part of the earliest version of the diet.

WHAT'S GOOD: The foods are healthy, though many popular foods are not permitted. The diet requires regular aerobic exercise, recommending walking no less than 45 minutes each day.

WHAT'S NOT SO GOOD: It's a very strict program, which can be difficult for many people to stick to. Also, you're eating a lot of fiber, which can produce excess gas. Portion sizes are not controlled.

THE COST: Just the cost of the book plus groceries.

protein power

THE SKINNY: This low-carb, high-protein, moderate-fat diet was a national best seller and has been compared to Atkins and the Zone. The major difference is portion control and awareness of calories—Protein Power doesn't permit dieters to enjoy unlimited amounts of proteins and fats. The focus is keeping your insulin level low.

WHAT'S GOOD: This diet can produce fast results, but the challenge is still keeping the weight off over time. The book discusses the importance of exercise, particularly resistance training. It is not extreme. It does not prescribe very low calories (like the Zone) or very low carb (like Atkins).

WHAT'S NOT SO GOOD: The first phase is very strict, with very low carbs, so it can be difficult to follow. Critics claim that the required calorie intake for some may be too low.

THE COST: Just the cost of the book plus groceries.

richard simmons

THE SKINNY: He's still around, and many dieters still like his sensible, exchange-oriented program coupled with lively, dance-oriented exercise. The program draws from the American Diabetic Association recommendations and is also based on motivating dieters to stay with the program.

WHAT'S GOOD: Simmons provides various tools to help with record keeping, such as the Food Mover. His upbeat motivation and emphasis on exercise can be very contagious.

WHAT'S NOT SO GOOD: Not everyone connects with Simmons's personal style of encouragement; if you don't like him, this won't work for you. If you dislike tracking or exchanges this may not be the plan for you.

THE COST: You can join his Clubhouse for twelve weeks for $20–$30, then pay $10/month to use the Web site and community. You get access to many online tools, but if you want hands-on help offline, you have to buy it through his store, which sells cookbooks, clothing, CDs, DVDs, the Food Mover (used to calculate servings), and much more.

the scarsdale diet

THE SKINNY: The doctor who created it is long gone, but the diet has stuck around, used by some as a jump start. It's a very low-calorie program with a very low-carb approach, not considered useful for long-term use.

WHAT'S GOOD: The diet tells you exactly what to eat and when, which some dieters prefer. Easy to dine out.

WHAT'S NOT SO GOOD: There is no snacking, and most meals are protein-heavy. The program includes herbal supplements, whose usefulness has been questioned. Exercise is not discussed, which may be a good thing based on the low-calorie nature of the program (700–1,000 calories per day).

THE COST: Just the cost of the book plus groceries.

shakes/liquid diets

THE SKINNY: This category includes all programs that encourage you to replace meals with a primarily liquid diet. You may remember that Oprah once lost sixty-seven pounds on a medically supervised diet using Optifast, but ultimately regained the weight. I used the same program, losing seventy pounds in three months and then regaining ninety in the following nine months. These days, most shake-centered diets are available over the counter in pharmacies.

WHAT'S GOOD: Shake diets can produce quick weight loss because they sharply reduce calorie intake.

WHAT'S NOT SO GOOD: It's very hard to eat out; most dieters bring their own shakes or eat earlier. It's easy to get quickly bored by the minimal choices. Also, you don't learn to control your food intake using regular foods.

THE COST: Costs vary depending on how many meals you replace with shakes. The average cost of each shake is between $1 and $3.

slim-fast

THE SKINNY: Originally, Slim-Fast was a shake-based diet plan, but now dieters can choose from snack and meal replacement bars, soups, juice drinks, and even pastas. You consume 1,200–1,500 calories each day (including one regular meal that you prepare or eat out) and are encouraged to get moderate exercise.

WHAT'S GOOD: There are many more flavor choices than there used to be, so dieters won't get bored as quickly. The products can be helpful to busy people who struggle to make time for food preparation. Online support is available at the company's Web site.

WHAT'S NOT SO GOOD: The products can be high in carbs and sugar, so they may not be as healthy as you'd like.

THE COST: The products vary in cost depending on where they're purchased and whether you buy individual items or multiples in big packages.

the sonoma diet

THE SKINNY: This Mediterranean-style diet plan was developed by a dietitian. The program encourages joy in eating and suggests that dieters emphasize ten power foods: almonds, bell peppers, blueberries, broccoli, grapes, olive oil, spinach, strawberries, tomatoes, and whole grains, plus a glass of wine each day.

WHAT'S GOOD: Three phases of weight loss get you off to a quick start (restrictive phase), then ease into a more manageable food plan (main weight loss phase), and then lifelong maintenance phase. Dieters are advised to practice portion control using plates of different sizes for different meals. The plan has a positive approach toward enjoyment as you lose weight.

WHAT'S NOT SO GOOD: It is not for those who don't enjoy spending time in the kitchen. If you're not a fan of wine, you may prefer a different approach. The diet does not have a strong exercise component.

THE COST: Just the cost of the cookbook plus groceries. The online program is $5 a week.

the south beach diet

THE SKINNY: This bestselling low-carb diet program asks dieters to eat reasonable portions of lean proteins (chicken, fish, lean beef) plus vegetables that are low on the glycemic index, moderate amounts of healthy fats (olive and canola oil, avocados, nuts), and small amounts of healthy carbs (whole grains, fruits). The promise, besides weight loss, is improved cardiovascular health (lower cholesterol and triglycerides). It's a three-phase program, moving from very restrictive to less so as you continue to follow the plan.

WHAT'S GOOD: The program is designed by a cardiologist and is considered the healthiest of the various low-carb programs available. Supports a healthy way of eating that is free of refined sugars and trans fats. The Web site provides dietitian support as well as additional recipes beyond what the books offer.

WHAT'S NOT SO GOOD: Some dieters find it hard to follow a program that limits carbohydrates. And some critics feel that the program's dependence on the glycemic index to determine food choices is controversial. No exercise guidelines.

THE COST: Just the cost of the cookbook(s) plus groceries. South Beach markets a number of its own food products, but using them is optional. The online program is about $6 a week.

the special k diet

THE SKINNY: You may have seen elated women dancing around their cereal bowls on TV. Originally based on the cereal alone, this diet plan now includes a product line of other food items and is being marketed as a legitimate option for weight loss. The Special K Challenge claims that if you eat two bowls a day plus follow their simple dietary guidelines, you will lose up to six pounds in two weeks.

WHAT'S GOOD: The products are nutritious, and the program is a basic low-calorie plan.

WHAT'S NOT SO GOOD: Dieters may find eating the same cereal and bars boring over time. Also, some critics claim it is lacking in balanced nutrition. There is no guidance in exercise.

THE COST: Just the cost of groceries.

sugar busters!

THE SKINNY: This low-carb program builds on the idea that many dieters should avoid not only refined foods but "white" products such as potatoes and pasta as well as vegetables such as corn and carrots.

WHAT'S GOOD: Eliminating refined foods is a good idea. Sugar Busters! also promotes exercise, recommending a cardio work-out four times per week. The book also offers a variety of no-sugar-added recipes and the Web site gives support through message boards.

WHAT'S NOT SO GOOD: Critics say there is no scientific research to support the elimination of many of these vegetables from a healthy diet.

THE COST: Just the cost of the book plus groceries.

suzanne somers—somersizing

THE SKINNY: The television star who started as Chrissy on *Three's Company* has built a big business based on this program, which involves food combining and suggests that metabolism can be boosted by the elimination of sugar and many carbs. Somers also suggests that dieters skip "funky foods" such as rice, alcohol, potatoes, whole milk, and nuts.

WHAT'S GOOD: You don't have to worry about portion control, as long as you combine correctly. She provides lots of tasty recipes in her books. She recommends thirty minutes of exercise a day, three days a week—it's low, but it's better than nothing.

WHAT'S NOT SO GOOD: Dairy is very restricted. There isn't much scientific basis for her theories. Very low calorie.

THE COST: The cost of the cookbooks plus purchase of her optional food products, including a sugar substitute.

take off pounds sensibly (tops)

THE SKINNY: Take Off Pounds Sensibly is a nonprofit, noncommercial support-group-based weight loss program that has been compared to Weight Watchers. Originally formed in 1948, TOPS claims to offer a "caring and supportive approach to weight control." It uses an exchange-based diet and offers a twenty-eight-day eating plan.

WHAT'S GOOD: The group offers nutrition and exercise advice to its more than two hundred thousand members worldwide. The support and incentives of the group have been found to be very motivational to members. Strong on motivation and positive reinforcement, a system of fun competitions and recognition. Members can even join retreats and rallies. Members' contributions also fund obesity research. It is comparatively inexpensive.

WHAT'S NOT SO GOOD: Chapters elect volunteer leaders from their membership. The program's identity may not appeal to younger dieters.

THE COST: $24 annually.

the usda diet

THE SKINNY: In 2005 the U.S. Department of Agriculture established new guidelines for optimum health: work out thirty to ninety minutes each day, eat less than 2,000 calories, and incorporate fruit, vegetables, grains, dairy, and meats into your diet as per the Food Guide Pyramid.

WHAT'S GOOD: This food plan is based on a lot of research and offers options for different age groups, including young people. The interactive Web site is very informative and extensive.

WHAT'S NOT SO GOOD: There's no place to go for inspiration or support, so once you read the info, you're essentially on your own. Also, it can be hard to eat the recommended number of servings and stay under 2,000 calories, which may be more than you need, depending on age, height, and weight.

THE COST: Just the cost of groceries.

volumetrics

THE SKINNY: Volumetrics is a weight loss program designed by Dr. Barbara Rolls, professor of nutrition at Pennsylvania State University. This diet promises to create a feeling of fullness after eating by advising dieters about the foods that are most satisfying, especially those that have a high percentage of water (most fruits and vegetables). These are foods that have a low ED (energy density) and thus have fewer calories for more volume.

WHAT'S GOOD: The recommended foods are generally healthy, and there are recipes to help dieters build menus using them. Exercise is encouraged, though not overly emphasized. Walking is highly recommended. This may be a good option for a volume eater.

WHAT'S NOT SO GOOD: Figuring out how to determine low–energy density foods can be confusing at best. The cost of more fresh foods and quality meats may run up the food bill.

THE COST: Just the cost of the book plus groceries.

the weigh down workshop

THE SKINNY: In this faith-based diet program founded by Gwen Shamblin, members attend weekly classes, watch an informative video, listen to supplied CDs at home, and fill out workbooks in an effort to draw on Christian teachings to support their long-term weight loss.

WHAT'S GOOD: Members are taught to eat when they feel physically hungry. Members find support in each other and the Bible and can also access online tools. Those looking for a faith-based program may find success here.

WHAT'S NOT SO GOOD: Dieters who have trouble determining physical hunger may have trouble with weight loss. There is little guidance from a nutritional or exercise standpoint. Group leaders are not nutritional experts.

THE COST: Members pay $103 plus shipping to receive CDs and workbooks and attend eight weeks of classes. Online costs are $300 annually for an individual, which includes classes, chatrooms, and materials.

weight watchers

THE SKINNY: This long-lived weight loss and maintenance organization continually tweaks its program to respond to member needs and the latest research. Members can attend weekly meetings, join At Work programs, or do it entirely online. Weight Watchers provides plenty of handouts and support materials to follow the program, for which members can choose to count points or eat off a list of core foods.

WHAT'S GOOD: The program is very flexible, and there are no forbidden foods. Anything with a nutrition label can be evaluated for its points value. Support is strong through leadership, members, and an excellent online site.

WHAT'S NOT SO GOOD: There is a learning curve initially, as members need to thoroughly understand the Good Health Guidelines and how to convert nutritional information to points. But information is well laid out and plentiful. Leaders go through a Weight Watchers training program but are not medical experts.

THE COST: There are a number of different plans, depending on which program you choose. The latest option is an unlimited monthly pass for about $40, which also gives access to e-tools. Meeting costs vary locally but range from $10 to $15 weekly plus the cost of groceries. There may also be an initial registration fee, which can range from $10 to $20. Weight Watchers products can be purchased in meeting rooms and at many stores, but their use is optional.

you on a diet

THE SKINNY: Created by two medical doctors, including Oprah's famed Dr. Oz, this book and program promise to help dieters focus on eliminating fat around the midsection by avoiding processed foods and choosing whole grains, fresh fruits, vegetables, and lean proteins. There is online support as well as a DVD (additional purchase) to offer help and inspiration.

WHAT'S GOOD: Exercise is an integral part of this program. The doctors do a good job of explaining the science, and there are lots of quizzes, "factoids," and myth busters throughout the text. The food plan emphasizes satiety—finding the foods that deliver satisfaction and reduce stomach fat.

WHAT'S NOT SO GOOD: There's a lot to think about and read through, but this did not seem to affect the book's speedy rise to best-seller status, as it is witty and engaging. The book does ask dieters to analyze their personal history, which may be more than some are prepared to do. Although reducing abdominal obesity is an excellent goal, specific spot reduction is, unfortunately, an impossibility in weight loss.

THE COST: Just the cost of the book plus groceries.

the zone diet

THE SKINNY: This low-carb diet asks dieters to eat 40 percent carbs, 30 percent lean protein, and 30 percent healthy fat. Dieters avoid unfavorable carbs such as brown rice, pasta, papaya, mango, banana, dry breakfast cereal, bread, bagels, tortillas, carrots, and all fruit juices. Your goal is to stay in the "Zone"—and control insulin.

WHAT'S GOOD: Weight loss can be rapid, and the recommended eating plan is good if you like protein.

WHAT'S NOT SO GOOD: Some critics have noted that it's hard to figure out what to eat. Also, eating low fiber may increase constipation, at least at first.

THE COST: Just the cost of the book plus groceries, unless you decide to use a Zone delivery service, which may cost $30 to $40 per day. Zone products are available but are optional.

is there one perfect diet for you?

Probably not. I'd bet there are several that might work for any one of us. One may appeal to you more than the others. That's the one to go for.

Don't be afraid to pick a diet that you've tried before, even if you didn't achieve long-term success on it. You're a different person now from the one who tried last time. This time, you're going to succeed because you are approaching the diet in a different way.

You have other resources available to you as you choose your diet plan. Have you noticed recently that a friend has lost weight and looks great? Ask her how she did it. Just keep in mind that whatever weight loss plan worked for your friend may not work for you—for instance, if your eating or cooking styles are very different. No matter what diets the two of you choose, you can provide motivational support to each other.

Also, check out your local bookstore or surf the Web. There's a tremendous amount of diet information on the Internet, including lots of message boards and reviews by people who've tried the programs.

Type a diet's name into your search engine and you'll be amazed at how many URLs come up. Or check page 122 for a list of my favorite Web sites. The content at many sites is not provided by experts with backgrounds in nutrition or medicine, so take what you read with a grain of salt. You have to distinguish between a review, expert information, and advertising copy. And sometimes it's not so easy to tell them apart.

Make time to talk with your doctor or health care provider before you start any weight loss plan. Taking charge of your health is an important step, and it's a good idea to share your expectations and concerns with a professional who already knows your medical history.

You've thought long and hard about what you like, what you eat, and what you need. Now it's time to make your choice!

set your goals

I used to hate football season. Actually, I adore football, it was just what the sportscasters used to say that bothered me. It was hard hearing them talk about the immense size of football players: "These guys are mass-s-s-sive. Weighing in at 250 pounds, this six-foot, five-inch linebacker could take out a tank. Don't get in his way, boys."

Hearing this, as I was driving along in my car, was devastating. I would just sit there and shake my head. I was a five-foot, six-inch female who outweighed these football players by one hundred pounds! Losing enough weight just to get down to the size of a football player, let alone a normal weight for a woman my size, seemed insurmountable. I thought, "It's impossible. I will never make it to goal. I will never, ever be thin."

was never much of a goal setter when it came to weight loss. I'm more of a dive-in-and-do-it kind of person. I didn't mind taking the time to write a grocery list or plan a meal or read weight loss material. It was directly related to what I was going to eat that day or how much weight I was going to lose that week.

But did I sit down and "plan realistic goals"? Nope. At that point, I would have said, "Are you kidding me? Here's a goal for you: *I want to lose this stupid weight!* Okay?"

How's that for goal setting?

But learning how to set goals and work toward them became a vital tool in my successful weight loss. So instead of asking you to stumble your way through that lesson the way I did, here's what I know now and wish I'd known then.

a *simple* goal-setting plan

When it's time for you to set your goals, think *SIMPLE:*

Specific
In Writing
Measurable
Possible
Limited in time
Enticing

specific

A general goal is "I need to lose some weight." It's vague, it's fuzzy, and it's likely to produce disappointing results. Instead, you want to specify exactly what you are looking to accomplish:

- "I'm going to work out at my gym on Monday nights, Wednesday mornings, and Saturday afternoons."

- "I'm going to spend an hour every Sunday chopping up vegetables for easy meal making during the week."

- "I'm going to go to my weight loss support group meeting every week, even if I'm afraid that I haven't lost any weight."

A specific goal is a promise you make to yourself that is as much a commitment as your required attendance at a meeting for your job or your appointment with your dentist (especially when the office charges a "no-show" fee). You *know* you have to show up!

> If you always do what you always did,
> you'll always get what you always got.

in writing

Goals that aren't in writing are just dreams or hopes for the future. But once you put them on paper they become a contract, a binding agreement with yourself. Otherwise, it's way too easy to forget what you said you would do. Your mind may deny it, but the evidence is before you.

Another great reason to write down your goals is to enjoy reviewing the process as time goes by. The earlier pages of your journal will make lively reading when you're a few months into your weight loss journey. You may revisit a page that describes a goal that once seemed so hard to reach—but now you're way past that number on the scale or lifting heavier weights!

measurable

Here's another way to keep your goals specific—make them *measurable.* Set a goal of eating a piece of fruit for a snack each afternoon, and you can check it off as you gobble it down! Instead of thinking, "I want to eat more fruit," use your numbers. If you're not happy with your recent blood tests, set a goal to drop thirty points of cholesterol. You'll *know* when you have accomplished it.

Most weight loss programs come with "ready-made" measurable goals—the numbers we want to see diminish on the scale. Remember to celebrate each milestone: That's part of the fun of measuring your success!

At the same time, don't forget to "measure" other accomplishments too—inches lost, walking pace quickened, number of stairs climbed without getting breathless.

possible

Goals need to be realistic. You may want to finish a 5K race as a goal for your first month, but if you've never run before, you're likely to be disappointed—and you'll hurt yourself by pushing your body too far, too fast.

> If you don't know where you're going,
> any road will take you.

Setting a new goal is an opportunity to stretch yourself, but it should also be attainable. It's better to set many smaller goals than to fix all your desires on one large one. Think of them as stepping-stones—an easy way to cross a wide, swiftly moving stream that would otherwise be too wide to cross. When I weighed in at 347 pounds, even the thought of losing 10 percent of my body weight—34 pounds—seemed an impossibility for me. It was way too far away. Instead, I aimed for interim successes: first 10 pounds, then 25, and then I longed to get out of the 300s into the 200s. If I'd thought about how long it was going to take to lose 200 pounds, I'd have thrown in the towel. Instead, I cheered each small win along the way.

In my meetings we celebrate with paper clips. I give dieters a paper clip for every pound they lose. As their chain gets longer and longer, it's a wonderful visual of how far they've come. They can't wait to get the next paper clip! It's not hard. It's just one pound. Two hundred pounds is the same thing, just one pound over and over again, two hundred times.

limited in time

Putting a time limit on a goal can be a powerful motivator, but I suggest you use time limits only on performance-based goals, not on getting specific weight loss results. People who say they are going to lose X number of pounds in X number of days often don't—and they get discouraged. You can only do the best you can to follow your program; you can't control what the scale or tape measure says on a given day.

SET A GOAL FOR ONE DAY: Tomorrow, I'm going to wear my new pedometer and try to cover at least ten thousand steps.

SET A GOAL FOR ONE WEEK: This week, I'm going to leave work on time at least three nights in order to go home and prepare dinner from scratch.

SET A GOAL FOR ONE MONTH: This month, I'm going to practice salsa dancing at home and go out with friends to a club to see how I do in public. (That was NOT one of my goals!)

SET A GOAL FOR ONE YEAR: This year, I'm going to plan an active vacation during which I will swim, ride a bike, and run in a triathlon. And I'm going to train by hitting the track, roads, and pool at least once a week each!

Use your time limits to keep yourself focused on all those great little victories. In the meantime, remember: As long as you reach your performance goals, the results *will* come.

enticing

This is the fun part—giving yourself rewards! I know that achieving your goals is a reward all by itself, but promising yourself a new pair of jeans or a manicure when you get there doesn't hurt!

If you are looking for ways to stay motivated and encouraged during your weight loss journey (and we all need them!), this is one of the best . . . and it really works. Just be sure your chosen reward isn't counterproductive—it makes no sense to celebrate a ten-pound loss by eating a whole large pizza.

Make a list of rewards you'd enjoy, from the latest hardcover mystery by your favorite author (don't wait for the paperback—buy it now to mark your conquest of the stair climber!) to something that will make your food or fitness routine more pleasurable—a fun kitchen tool or a cool case for the iPod you listen to at the gym.

I remember the first goal-setting experience I had at a Weight Watchers meeting one Thursday morning. My leader, Beth, gave each of us an index card and asked us to write three goals for the New Year. She said they didn't have to be weight-loss oriented, but they did have to be *realistic* and *positive.* I accomplished all three goals and I still have that index card today.

Setting goals becomes easier and faster the more you do it. Goal setting should be fun, not stressful. Keep your goals positive, thinking of them as wishes made real, a step that can get you where you want to go. Write them into your journal or planner. Here's a page from the one I created. Photocopy it if you like, or just use it as a guide when creating a format that works best for your needs.

Thoughts:

_____

_____

_____

_____

_____

_____

_____

_____

_____

Activity	Time/Distance	Intensity

My food goal for tomorrow is:

_____

_____

My activity goal for tomorrow is:

_____

_____

3

plan

I do a lot more traveling now than I used to, mostly to places I've never been before, for speaking engagements and for TV. In my office, I keep a folder for each new destination. Inside, I put all the pertinent information: individuals to contact, MapQuest directions or flight information and boarding passes, phone numbers, whatever I may need for the journey. When the time comes for me to leave, all I have to do is grab the folder and follow the directions. Sometimes there is an unforeseen glitch, but for the most part, getting from point A to point B is easy. Piece of cake. I learned all of this organization the hard way.

One time, I was invited to speak at an all-day seminar in New Jersey, about four hours from home. For some reason, I thought I knew where I was going and how to get there. Disorganized and running late, I threw everything into the car at the last minute. I quickly discovered I needed help—and I made it on time only because Mark talked me through the directions by cell phone the entire way.

Coming home was another story altogether. I didn't call home for help because I figured I'd just retrace my steps. It wasn't that easy. By the time I hit the Jersey shore—having driven many miles in the opposite direction from where I needed to go—I realized just how lost I really was. It was nearly midnight and I was having trouble staying awake. I thought, if only I had taken the extra time up front to plan my trip and make sure I understood the directions, I could have saved so much time, energy, money, and wear and tear on my body.

t's exactly the same with our diets. When we start any kind of diet regimen, we want to think *less* about food, to put it out of our minds. The problem is, nothing could be less helpful! Of course, it depends to some degree on what diet you choose to follow, but most people need time to learn the program well. My advice to anyone who longs to be *finally thin*:

The amount of time and effort you put in, especially in the beginning, is directly proportional to your ultimate success. Don't *take* the time, *make* the time.

In fact, I warn anyone starting to follow a new food plan that they need to be planning their food, thinking about food, shopping for food, and learning new ways to cook their food more during those first few weeks than they have ever before!

That's the difference between a temporary, quick-fix diet and a permanent, reach-your-goal lifestyle—*time.* How can something become a fixture, an important part of who you are without a real investment of time? When you begin a new career, it can take years to develop the skills you need to succeed and advance in it. The learning curve can be enormous. Think about how much work it takes to become proficient when you're learning to play a musical instrument. There's a big difference between getting noise out of a cello and sounding like the world-renowned cellist Yo-Yo Ma. Well, plucking the strings and being satisfied with some screeches is yo-yo dieting, and playing a concerto the way Yo-Yo Ma does is making your diet your lifestyle.

If you take nothing else away from this book, I urge you to plan and prepare your meals. Without planning your daily menus, your success will be a gamble at best. You *may* have what you need in your cupboards when you get home . . . or you may not. You *may* have enough points or calories or carbs left for the evening snack you crave . . . or you may not. If you "mess up," you *may* just decide to throw in the towel and start again tomorrow.

Lack of planning equals deprivation, and deprivation equals yo-yo dieting. You've already done that—and don't want to do it again.

Planning what you're going to eat does take time, but it will take less time the more you do it. Getting "good" at planning is a gift you can give yourself, and it's a gift that will last you forever, a long-term, risk-free investment in the rest of your life.

what planning requires

To make a successful meal plan for most diet programs, you have to know four key elements:

1. *Know the **quantity** requirements.* Whether you're counting points or carbs or calories or exchanges, you need to know exactly what you are allowed—each day, each week, however the plan is designed.

2. *Know the **nutritional** requirements.* If you're allowed 1,400 calories per day, and you eat 1,400 calories' worth of waffles, you won't lose weight and keep it off *or* be healthy. Besides advising you about the quantity of food to eat, most healthy meal plans provide you with a list of how much to eat from each food group.

3. *Know your **time** requirements.* Some diet plans stipulate *when* you should eat and how often. Even if your chosen diet doesn't specify eating times, I recommend that you plan to eat a meal or a light snack at least every three hours. This keeps your metabolism chugging along, your sugar levels more even, and extreme hunger at bay—one of the most important reasons for eating at regularly scheduled times.

4. *Know your **personal** requirements.* Do you go to the movies every Friday night? Have dinner with the girls each Saturday? Really want those egg rolls when your office orders Chinese takeout? If you keep these kinds of "facts of life" in mind when you plan your weekly menus, you can usually fit in what you want to eat—*without* guilt, *without* fear, *without* running out.

I've used a variety of food-planning and -tracking tools during my "diet career." Here's one of my favorites: Take an index card and write down BREAKFAST, LUNCH, DINNER, and SNACKS. Write exactly what you are going to have under each heading, *including* the calories or points or carbs for each item. The card should look like you've already eaten it—completely filled in. Then just check it off as you go. The work is all done ahead of time.

These days, you've got lots of great planning choices, so opt for whatever feels comfortable and works for you: an index card, a small memo book, a special weight loss journal, your iPhone, or a Web site that allows you to track your eating online.

Successful journaling looks different for everyone. Some people write carefully and with lots of details; others use abbreviations to symbolize dishes or foods they eat frequently.

Don't just do it and toss it, either. *Save* your daily food journals on your computer, in a three-ring binder, in a recipe card box—whatever works. I punched a hole in the upper left-hand corner of each card and kept them all on a small ring. As they started to accumulate I could flip through the days I had already used. Sometimes I'd just grab a card and reuse it. Other times, I would look back at the cards for ideas, especially if I felt I was in a meal-planning rut and my meals were getting too routine or boring. Try what sounds best to you. Before you know it, you will have created your own personalized food plan.

Unique to you. Perfect for you.

hate to plan?

If your day's food is planned out and you know what's coming next, your rate of success will increase dramatically. But if you really hate to plan, why not start with something manageable? For week one, make it your goal to plan out three days' worth of different meal plans. Then, using leftovers and reinventing a few things, you can switch it up a little here and there and stretch those nine meals into plans for seven days.

For the next week, add two or three more daily plans. By the end of ten weeks you'll have enough unique, individual meal plans to provide you with a different menu each day for a month. And remember, these are all meals *you've* chosen and prepared and enjoy.

With the exception of special occasions, most people don't need more than thirty different breakfasts, lunches, and dinners. But to keep it fun and exciting, I'm always trying new recipes and creating new daily plans. It's what I do, what I enjoy. Find what works for you and *do it*!

Here is a copy of the planner page (see page 102) I designed for my own weight loss planning and journaling. Use it if you like it, or create your own.

Plan what you will do.
Then do what you have planned.

Day: _____   Target Intake: _____

Breakfast
_____ | _____
_____ | _____
_____ | _____

Lunch
_____ | _____
_____ | _____
_____ | _____

Dinner
_____ | _____
_____ | _____
_____ | _____

Snacks
_____ | _____
_____ | _____

Total Intake: _____

Weight: _____

+ / −: _____

☐ Fat
☐ ☐ Fruit
☐ ☐ ☐ Dairy
☐ ☐ ☐ ☐ Veggies
☐ ☐ ☐ ☐ ☐ Protein
☐ ☐ ☐ ☐ ☐ ☐ Carbs
☐ ☐ ☐ ☐ ☐ ☐ ☐ Waters

Use the check boxes to ensure that you are eating a well-balanced diet.

Note: Individual diet plans may vary.

be prepared
(it's not just a motto for boy scouts)

Part of planning is being prepared. There's no point to planning your meals if you're not able to make and eat what you put down on paper.

If I plan to serve turkey patties for dinner, I have to make sure my meat is defrosting in the refrigerator before I go to work. If I'm going to have popcorn for a snack and I won't be home again before snack time, I pop it and throw the bag in the back of the car. (Why don't I keep it up front? I know myself well enough to know I'd chow down on it way before I was hungry if it were sitting right next to me!)

terrific time-saving preparation tips

We all have days when we arrive home exhausted and ravenous. For those occasions, you'll be so glad you prepared extra servings of meals ahead of time and froze them for easy reheating. Here are some good ways to make this happen:

1. When you come home from the grocery store, weigh and measure bulk-packaged foods and package them individually.

2. Before freezing poultry, wash and add marinades; before freezing meats, divide them into portions and add marinades, rubs, or seasonings.

3. Stop at a local restaurant or grocery store salad bar for a quick and easy salad or to buy some cut-up veggies for a stir-fry. Steam broccoli florets or throw a mixture of peppers, mushrooms, and onions into a large frying pan with nonfat cooking spray and light teriyaki sauce. (I love Kikkoman in a packet—just add water. It's *so* good!)

4. Regularly go through your cupboards, refrigerator, and pantry and make sure you're well stocked on grocery staples that help you stick to your diet. And pitch all "red-light foods" (foods that you find way too hard to resist—and can put a red light in your diet's success).

5. Don't let yourself run out of the fresh fruits and veggies that you need each day. But just in case, keep some canned and/or frozen ones on hand.

the ten steps to a finally thin life

6. Keep a nonperishable snack in your glove compartment, office desk, or purse for emergencies. Unexpected delays can ignite your hunger for a high-fat, sugary "reward."

7. Write out a detailed grocery shopping list as you plan your meals. It will ultimately save you time, money, and temptation at the grocery store!

Just to help you in your planning, here's a list I love—tasty snacks that you can enjoy for 70 calories or less:

standby snack list (70 calories or less):

- ½ Kim's Light Bagel with 1 teaspoon whipped cream cheese
- Campbell's Soup at Hand soups—especially Chicken with Mini Noodles
- 1¼ cups vegetable juice with two celery stalks
- 1 cup sugar-free pudding (any flavor) made with nonfat milk
- 1-ounce bag Lays Light Potato Chips
- 1 medium apple or orange
- 1¼ cups berries
- 6 ounces sugar-free light yogurt with 4 tablespoons berries
- ¾ cup light cranberry juice mixed with ½ cup seltzer
- 1 cup raw celery and carrots with ¼ cup Party Shrimp Dip (see recipe on page 214)
- 2 cups steamed cauliflower with spray butter and 2 teaspoons fat-free Parmesan
- 1 piece part-skim string cheese
- 1¼ cups Hot Cocoa Mix (see recipe on page 189)

If you fail to plan, you plan to fail.

- 5 large shrimp with 1 tablespoon ketchup, 1 teaspoon horseradish, and ½ teaspoon lemon juice mixed well.

- ⅓ cup low-fat ice cream in a flat-bottom cone

- 1 medium hard-boiled egg

- 1 entire package prepared sugar-free Jell-O with 4 tablespoons fat-free Cool Whip

- 1 cup Cream of Broccoli Soup (see recipe on page 240)

Remember, you don't have to figure it *all* out in the first week. Learn the basics right away. Make up a week's worth of daily plans to follow. Rotate them and change them up a little. Try out some new "lite" grocery items here and there, a few at a time. Be willing to try new things, and before you know it you'll have expanded your world of food choices dramatically.

make over your environment

You arrive home after a busy day at work. It's late. You've carefully followed your diet all day, but now you're starving. What can you throw together that's quick and light? You check the cupboards and find an old box of macaroni and cheese—and plenty of pasta. Hmm, that mac & cheese should have been pitched weeks ago when you started your diet, and because you ate lunch out today, even the pasta has too many calories and carbs. You need something really light and filling.

What about that bean chili recipe? That's quick, and you can have a lot of it for just a few calories. You check the cabinets—oh, too bad, you don't have all the ingredients. Your stomach growls as you open the refrigerator and stare at the empty shelves. You're hungry, tired, and stuck. The mac & cheese looks like the only option. You eat it, but you don't enjoy a mouthful. You know it's high in calories, fat, and sodium. You had to eat something, but after all that hard work, why did you leave yourself without any healthy choices?

S uccess in dieting takes action. Signing up for a support group and reading diet books doesn't mean that change is going to happen automatically. You have to be proactive and *DO IT*!

Start by purging your home. Go into all of the cabinets and get rid of everything that represents real temptation for you. As a mom, I like to keep some snacks in the house for my kids, but there are some things I still can't have around. I can buy Vienna Fingers cookies and never think of them once I've put my groceries away. But I can't have Oreos in my house.

My kids don't care which cookies. *I do.* If I gave them a choice, they'd probably pick the Oreos, too, but if I don't buy them, they don't miss them. It's a lesson I've learned over time—if I buy a package of Oreos, I know who I'm really buying them for—and who is likely to gobble them down!

Anything, even good-for-you low-fat products, can cause trouble for someone on a weight loss program. One of my members chooses not to buy the low-fat chocolate fudge bars that she loves so much. When a member asked her why, she answered, "I once bought a box of six—and I ate them all in one day. Even though I stayed within my points, I knew it was unhealthy behavior." Bravo! She occasionally splits a package with two other members. They each go home with two bars and are very happy.

Does that mean that you can never have these foods? *Absolutely not!* Just not now. In the beginning I got rid of a lot of things that I have in my home today without even thinking about it. (But I never allow cake into the house in any way, shape, or form. Still can't do it. And I'm okay with that.)

When Alan, Andrew, and I go to the grocery store, I often plan in two points for our little snack cake favorites. There are six one-point treats in the box and each of us eats two as we shop. They're happy. I'm happy. We pay with an empty box and smile at the knowing looks from the cashier. I'm not depriving myself. I am making a smart decision about what I can and can't handle.

Make sure you stock your home with what you need to do the job you've chosen. Whatever it takes to keep you on track, consider it an investment in better health . . . and happiness.

Here's a checklist of kitchen tools to help get you started:

☐ Nonstick cookware/bakeware

☐ Light cookbooks

☐ Calorie- and/or carb-counting books

☐ Trackers/planners/food diaries

- ☐ Grocery lists

- ☐ Measuring spoons and cups

- ☐ Electronic food scale

- ☐ Blender

- ☐ Sugar substitutes

- ☐ Nonfat cooking spray

- ☐ Sugar-free gum/breath mints

I know how busy everyone is. I have my plate full as well. But wanting to lose weight is not enough to make it happen. So get busy. Remember, the more prepared you are, the less willpower you'll need! Making over your home environment is one of the best ways to avoid temptation and "stay on the wagon."

Prepare your home for your weight loss journey. Go shopping and fill your fridge, cupboards, and freezer with healthy foods that *you* find appealing. Here's my most recent Guilt-Free Grocery List. Carry it with you when you shop—and you'll be amazed at how many delicious options you've got!

Because new products hit the stores every month, I revise this list frequently. You can find the most up-to-date version of this list on my Web site, kimbensen.com.

This is a list to help get you started, but now the best thing you can do is to choose the light products that are *your* favorites. I've zeroed in on lots of possibilities, but you're going to need to do some scouting of your own. Start by reading labels. It can be frustrating and even overwhelming, but once you get the hang of it and know what to look for (and what to avoid), you're ready to shop.

the package says "light," but is it?

Think how easy dieting would be if you had cupboards full of delicious light snacks, an abundance of fresh fruits and veggies in your fridge, and all the ingredients you needed to make that lovely new casserole from *Cooking Light* magazine!

Yes, and wouldn't it be nice if the Fat-Free Fairy Godmother (FFFG) could make it all magically appear in your house—and remove those Oreos while she was at it!

Well, turn around three times and grab your wand because *you* are your own FFFG! Shopping for weight loss takes time and know-how. Oh yeah, and money. But it doesn't have to blow your budget and it's less costly than being unhealthy! The following list of do's and don'ts to filling a grocery cart will help you stay on track all week long.

DO: Shop with an itemized list. Keeping a running list will save you time and money. You'll pass by all those tempting snacks because, well, they're *not on your list*!

DON'T: Shop on an empty stomach. Or, if you have to, grab a container of grape tomatoes, a bag of baby carrots, or some other healthy snack to nibble on as you roll up and down the aisles. (Don't forget to pay for it when you get to the register!)

DO: Try new food items. If you're purchasing the same things all the time, you're likely to get bored—and boredom can be death to a diet!

DON'T: Shop for foods that are out of season. Seasonal produce is more affordable, much tastier, and fresher, too.

DO: Shop for reduced-fat products and foods lower in sugar. Even slight changes in foods you eat regularly can add up to a big savings in calories.

DON'T: Buy "red-light foods" because you fear that you are depriving your family members. They want you to be healthy and successful on your diet. If you can't handle it, they don't need it.

DO: Read those labels. It's an important part of making wise food choices. If you have trouble understanding nutrition labels, you're not alone! The next section of this chapter will give you a crash course. You'll get the hang of it quickly, I promise!

Don't become discouraged when a shopping trip that used to take thirty minutes now takes you close to an hour. You'll soon pick up the pace, once you know what you need and where to find it.

It may feel like visiting a brand-new grocery store. In the beginning, just finding the milk can be frustrating! But within a few weeks, you're in the groove and can whiz through the aisles finding everything on your list.

That's how it is with *healthy* grocery shopping. You may be tempted to grab "the usual" because it's easier to find what you've always purchased, but be patient. Before long, shopping for healthy products will be as effortless as food shopping ever was.

let's talk about labels

You're walking down the aisles of the grocery store, innocently minding your own business, when your eye is drawn to the marketing on every package: Low-carb! Fat-free! Heart-healthy! Organic! No sugar added!

Over here! I'm healthy! Pick me!

It's hard to ignore these entreaties from the fronts of all those packages. They're designed to get your attention and persuade you to buy. But don't succumb so easily. Not until you've checked out the label on the back.

The box may say "lite," but that doesn't mean it's light by the standards of someone who's trying to lose weight. The truth is, although food manufacturers cannot lie to you about the nutrition facts or ingredients in their products, they *can* easily mislead you. No! Really?!

Reading and understanding a nutrition label is really pretty easy if you know what you're looking for.

"light" or "lite"

For a product to be labeled "light" or "lite," it has to contain *one-third fewer calories or half the fat or half the sodium of the regular verson*. It can have less fat and fewer calories than the original but still have a *ton* of fat and calories, depending on what the original product was.

"low calorie"

Low calorie simply means 40 calories or less per serving. Again, watch the serving size. Some of them are pretty unrealistic.

"low fat"

The FDA gives a low-fat rating to a product if it has 3 grams of total fat or less per serving. For fish, poultry or meat, a food labeled lean means it has less than 10 grams of total fat per 3-ounce serving. Extra lean means it has less than 5 grams of total fat per 3-ounce serving.

"fat free"

The FDA allows a product to be called "fat free" if it has *less than half a gram of fat per serving*. That doesn't mean there is *no* fat in the product. "Calorie-free" cooking sprays have a whopping 350 to 600-plus servings in one can (depending on the brand). Each teeny-tiny serving is techni- cally calorie free simply because the serving size is a lightning-quick one-third-of-a-second spray. (I'm quick in the kitchen, but even I don't have reflexes like that!)

Actually, according to the Pam Web site, a one-second spray has 7 calories and a two-second spray has 15. Try coating your frying pan in less than two seconds, I dare you! Still, it's a lot less than using cooking oil. Just try not to drench your pans and food with the stuff—and your hips will love you for it.

"zero trans fats"

This is a scary one, in my opinion. Trans fats came from the process of turning liquid vegetable oil into a solid by adding hydrogen to it. Its pur- pose was to increase the shelf life of processed foods. That's what makes Crisco and margarine what they are today. It is fake fat that can raise your LDLs and lower your HDLs, and that's not good. Packaging doesn't always tell you what you want to know about this additive. Don't trust a product's claim of zero trans fats *and* don't even trust the Nutrition Facts label on this one. Here you have to always read the ingredients list.

If the words *partially hydrogenated* appear in it at all, then the food *does* contain trans fats. Thanks to current labeling guidelines, any food that contains 0.5 grams or less of a nutrient can be listed as zero grams on the Nutrition Facts label. This may seem insignificant, but it does add up. If the serving size of a box of cookies is one cookie and that cookie contains 0.5 grams of trans fats—well, how many of you eat only one cookie? Think about all the trans fats you (and your kids) may be consuming from that box of "zero trans fats" cookies. *Yikes!* According to the latest research, there is no safe level of trans fat consumption, so beware of foods with any in them.

step-by-step label reading

1. Start at the top with Servings Per Container. If the Servings Per Container is one, all the numbers listed below are for everything in that package. If, however, the Servings Per Container is two or more, and you plan on eating the entire package, you're going to have to multiply all the numbers (calories, fat, etc.) by the number of servings per container.

2. Check the number of calories per serving. If the package has four servings, and each serving has 120 calories, the whole box has 480 calories.

   Here's a great example: Campbell's Chicken & Stars Condensed Soup and Campbell's Chicken & Stars Soup at Hand.

   Both soups taste great and have 70 calories per serving. However, if you read carefully you will see that there is one serving in the Soup at Hand soup (70 calories), but 2.5 servings in the condensed soup (70 calories × 2.5). Therefore, if you were to eat the entire can of condensed Chicken & Stars soup, you would be getting 175 calories.

3. The next nutrients—fat, cholesterol, sodium—are ones you want to limit.

4. The last nutrients listed—fiber, vitamins, calcium, iron—are ones you want to make sure you get enough of.

5. Confused by all those percentages in the right-hand column? They refer to "percent daily value" (%DV) based on the government's recommendation for key nutrients. They're a bit trickier to interpret, and no, they are not supposed to add up to 100 percent. The FDA bases these percentages on a 2,000-calorie-a-day diet. If you don't know how many calories a day you're eating, you can still use the %DV as a reference point to figure out whether a food is high or low in a nutrient. Five percent or less is low, and a good range for nutrients that you want to limit (fat, saturated fat, cholesterol, and sodium), and 20 percent or more is high—a good range for things you want to eat plenty of (fiber, calcium, and vitamins).

Understanding the Nutrition Label

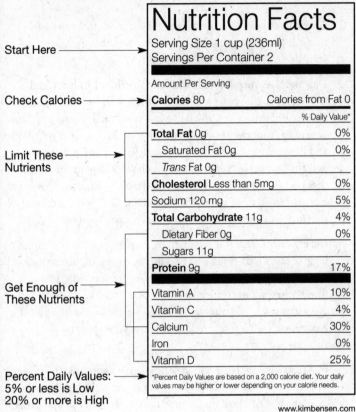

Start Here

Check Calories

Limit These Nutrients

Get Enough of These Nutrients

Percent Daily Values: 5% or less is Low 20% or more is High

Nutrition Facts

Serving Size 1 cup (236ml)
Servings Per Container 2

Amount Per Serving

Calories 80	Calories from Fat 0
	% Daily Value*
Total Fat 0g	0%
Saturated Fat 0g	0%
Trans Fat 0g	
Cholesterol Less than 5mg	0%
Sodium 120 mg	5%
Total Carbohydrate 11g	4%
Dietary Fiber 0g	0%
Sugars 11g	
Protein 9g	17%
Vitamin A	10%
Vitamin C	4%
Calcium	30%
Iron	0%
Vitamin D	25%

*Percent Daily Values are based on a 2,000 calorie diet. Your daily values may be higher or lower depending on your calorie needs.

www.kimbensen.com
Source3: www.cfsan.fda.gov

Love those "calorie-free," "fat-free" products? Me too! But each container can contain up to 900 calories and 90 grams of fat. Yikes! (If you're a Fat-Free ReddiWip mouth squirter—you know who you are!) That, too, is for a very small serving. If you gobble down more than one serving (there are forty servings in a can), then you *will* be getting about 200 calories per can.

Remember that the FDA allows "fat free" status for a product that has less than a half a gram of fat *per serving.* Hey, I think it's still worth the squirt. Just make sure you squirt *responsibly.*

clean up your environment 1—2—3

1. *Get rid of all your "red-light foods."* Those foods that call your name as you walk past the kitchen. The ones that nudge you in your sleep. *Get them out of the house!*

2. *Do a swap.* As you clean out your cupboards, refrigerator, and freezer, replace high-fat and sugary foods with lighter choices. Choose ones you think you'll like and continually reevaluate your selections. Your taste buds and cravings often change as your body and lifestyle are altered. But make sure you are eating *only* products that you enjoy. I eat way too much salad to pour on a dressing that I don't like. To stick with my food plan, I've got to enjoy every bite! The good news is, new light products arrive on the market all the time—so keep looking when you visit your market!

3. *Get organized.* This is no small thing. Remember that one of the biggest reasons diets fail *isn't* because we can't handle temptation, it's because we don't take time to plan or prepare. With that in mind, you want to create an environment at home, at work, and away that supports your goal of losing weight and keeping it off. Ask yourself what you can do to increase your chances of success.

   - Are you going to use a food scale when you prepare your meals? (Please say yes!) Is it currently buried under the holiday dishes in the black hole of the corner cupboard? Get it out and make room for it. I recommend that you set it right on the counter as a reminder to *use* it.

   - Where are your light cookbooks and other diet resources? How about your calorie counters, your carb finders? Do you have them all where they should be—right next to the blank grocery list? Do you have your food plan for the week made out? Keep it in a visible spot and make sure you've got a pencil or pen to update and edit it.

Thin begins in the grocery store.

- If you plan on having food delivered, do you have the order number saved on your speed dial? Make sure you order in time!

- Are you all set to use online tracking? Have you signed up and do you know your password? Bookmarked your page? Or are you going to use a tracking bracelet? Journal? Index cards?

Come on—get going and get organized. You'll be so glad you did!

But wait, home isn't your only environment. There's the office, the car, even your best friend's house and your in-laws'. Think about how much time you spend at these places and figure out what you'll need when you are there. Creating an environment that supports your weight loss goals is not just a good idea—it's really the only way to exercise control over what you eat away from home. By putting thought and time into preparing the places where you spend hours at a time, you can avoid many temptations and keep your eyes on the prize!

gather your support

After dieting for just over a year, I had lost nearly a hundred pounds. My husband was so proud of me, so excited for me. Mark's always loved me, no matter what size I was, and he's seen them all, from a slim 6 to an almost-impossible-to-find 6X. He would do anything to support my new healthy lifestyle, knowing just how much it meant to me. Case in point:

We went to Massachusetts during the summer to visit my favorite aunt and other relatives. We got there and piled into the kitchen. The whole family was hungry after the long road trip, including me. But I had planned ahead. I had called Tina and knew she was having a vegetable lasagna. Yum!

When we got there, the aroma of that delicious lasagna filled the kitchen. "It smells wonderful, Auntie. I'm starved!" I gave her a bear hug. "It's premade vegetable lasagna, sweetie. We've had it before. It's really delicious," she said. I asked if I could check out the packaging and read the nutritional label. What a shocker! I'm sure it was delicious. The fat and calorie content were through the roof.

I had only a limited number of points left that day and would be able to eat only a few bites if I wanted to stay within my limit. Mark saw the look of dismay on my face and gave me an encouraging smile. Before anyone realized he'd gone out, he was back— with a loaded grocery bag. He had headed down to a little market and picked up a big prepared salad and grilled chicken. I was able to sit down and enjoy a wonderfully satisfying, low-calorie dinner *with my family. I hadn't thought to do this for myself. It took someone determined to support me to provide just what I needed. Thanks, babe!*

S omeone, somewhere, at some point will see how desperate I am and save me. If it gets bad enough, someone will step in and do something.

I never said it out loud, never really formulated the thought, but I wished for it and felt it with all my heart. Did you ever feel that way, as if you were sinking, drowning, going down for the last time? Have you prayed that at some point someone would see your plight and help you?

If you have, join the club. There are lots of us out there.

Sometimes we long so much and so deeply for this "savior" to come, we lose sight of an important truth: *No one can do it for us.* It finally dawned on me that if I was going to be saved, I was going to have to be the one taking action. Finally, I got busy doing what I had to do. But I knew I couldn't do it without support.

There is a big difference between being *saved* and being *supported.* One isn't going to happen; the other one can make all the difference between success and failure.

my support team

My friend Cathy and I joined Weight Watchers at the same time. So from the start, we had each other as well as our leader, Beth, to guide us. We also had the meeting's other members to commiserate with and share ideas. That was my first line of support.

The rest of my family was there for me as well. Every week, after my weigh-in, I would buckle up my two little boys and hop in my minivan, and even before I started the car and left the Weight Watchers parking lot, I would whip out my cell phone and call my mom and my sister. My mom was only one town away, but my sister was all the way out in Minnesota. First Mom, then Heather, would hoot and holler and cheer and

A cord of three strands is not easily broken.

make me feel wonderful. They knew how much my dream meant and would join with me in celebrating. There were weeks, too, when they provided a listening ear when the scale had been unkind.

When I got home, my older two kids always wanted to know how I was doing. Each week, Aleeta took a picture of me in my weigh-in outfit and Adam gave me a big hug, telling me how proud he was. Their pride and interest in what I was doing motivated me to keep doing it. Even my extended family all exclaimed over my progress. Today my brother-in-law Alan jokes that he heads up the Kim Bensen fan club. If my Aunt Tina had charged me for all the hours she spent in "encouragement counseling" on the phone I'd be bankrupt and she'd be set for life! Love you, Auntie! I depended so much on my support system—and I'm so grateful for the opportunity to tell them so!

After I reached goal, amazing support continued to come from my friends and family. My best friend's husband, Dan, was so proud of me that he insisted on giving me one dollar for each pound I had lost so I could buy new clothes! *Wow! Two hundred twelve dollars!* (Thanks, Dan.)

Then support started coming from my new employer, Weight Watchers International, Inc., as they sent me to leadership training, made me a success story on their Web site, and opened up the world of online support to me. There I met other members and leaders who were looking for new recipes and products and struggling with the same daily issues I was. As a leader, meeting weekly with my wonderful members gave me back far more than I could ever have given them. Today, my good friend and now co-worker Peter is a constant source of encouragement and accountability . . . thanks, P!

what about you?

Who will *you* talk to when you feel lonely, disappointed, or discouraged during your weight loss journey? Not everyone has my large, crazy family. Some may even have friends and family members who exhibit the opposite of support—sabotage. So where will *your* support come from?

Well, take a moment to think about what real support looks like and feels like. I think the best support people have a listening ear and a big shoulder. They provide big bear hugs when we've had a bad week—even if they're miles away. Some days, supporters need to be there to cheer us on; other days, to give us a kick in the pants—and remind us what we wanted when we began.

Support comes in many different forms, and sometimes it comes from a source you don't expect. Start by thinking about what kind of support *you* need.

- Do you prefer to do most activities with one close friend? Then try to find a buddy to partner with as you both lose weight.

- Are you the kind of person who needs one-on-one encouragement, someone to "stay on your case"? You may do best to enlist a personal trainer or nutrition coach who will check in regularly and give you specific direction.

- Do you know the ropes but need fresh ideas to keep you going when the road seems so long? You may choose to lurk on an online bulletin board, knowing that you've got a large number of unseen friends who may feel just as you do—and are up at 1 a.m.!

- Part of your support team may be an organization such as your employer or church or your town's adult education programs.

Enlisting some kind of support, whether you opt for family, friends, a weight loss counselor, or an online chat room, is essential for mastering long-term weight loss. But everyone's needs are different. Your support team needs to be unique—a system that works specifically for you. Remember that your needs may change along the way, especially when the journey stretches in time. At the beginning, you may want to share your experiences with only a close friend, choosing not to speak up in your support group meeting. But a few months down the road, yours may be the first hand raised when your leader asks the group for ideas to help a new member!

Some members of your support team may never know they're on your list. It may include the server at your neighborhood café who remembers to bring skim milk for your coffee, and your aunt and uncle in Ohio who keep you in their prayers. All successful people will tell you about the supporters who helped them get there: Almost nobody does it alone.

We often feel guilty when we ask others to go out of their way for us, alter behaviors for us, give up foods they enjoy having around. We also tend to show our love in food. We see holiday treats and new cookies and favorite snacks and we want to bring joy to those we love.

Fact: No one, even active teenagers, is going to benefit from high-calorie, high-fat junk food. Even our kids won't always be active teenagers. Setting good habits now is a gift you can give them. *Fact:* No

> As iron sharpens iron,
> so one friend sharpens another.

one who cares about you is going to mind making behavioral changes to help you on such an important venture. Would you mind helping them? *Fact:* Those who do mind will get over it. If not, it's their problem, not yours.

sign them up

Don't wait until you're under way to gather your support team together. That would be like waiting until you're two hundred miles down the road to ask the gas station mechanic to check your oil! Here's a list of support suggestions. Add to it, *be imaginative,* and be open to what different people in your life can offer:

- Ask a friend to join you on your diet. Find a friend who is starting the same program the week you are, and buddy up. Just make sure that your success is not tied in to your friend's. Encourage each other, but don't be pulled down if he or she gets off track.

- Explain your plan to your kids, your spouse, or your roommates. Tell them what foods you would rather not have in the house for now.

- Enlist volunteers to help put leftovers away and do the dinner dishes so you can get *out of the kitchen faster.*

- Ask close friends to check in with you each week and see how you're doing.

- Encourage loved ones to put their snacks away when they're done nibbling. *Out of sight* may not be totally out of mind, but it *helps!*

- Ask sympathetic co-workers to keep their goodies out of the community kitchen or to store them unseen inside containers in the fridge. If this isn't possible or is too hard to manage, consider buying a dorm-type fridge for you and colleagues who want to focus on healthy eating at work.

- Invite your kids to join you on a bike ride or walk before or after dinner. The reward is not only increased fitness but more you-and-me time with them!

- Plan to go grocery shopping with your spouse so that the two of you can work together to find the healthiest selections.

- Ask your server to give you the inside scoop on lighter menu selections *and* don't be afraid to ask for special preparations or substitutions. Remember, this is a health issue, not just picky eating. Tell yourself, "I'm allergic to that. I break out in fat!"

- Talk to your doctor about your weight loss plan and discuss any specific concerns you need to focus on.

- E-mail your goals to a friend and ask him or her to send them back to you every so often. We sometimes forget what we felt when we started out, and it can be great to revisit those feelings!

- If you're having difficulty sticking to your menus, ask a friend if you can e-mail him or her your food plan every morning to keep you accountable.

- Ask your trainer (or your teenager, as I did) to take before and as-you-go photos to keep you motivated. Don't keep them in a drawer, either. Paste one on the cover of your weight loss journal if you think it will help. Some of us are motivated more from "good" pictures, so if you've got one from a time when your weight was healthier, use that instead!

- Your home isn't the only place that you want to make "diet friendly." Ask co-workers and friends for their cooperation. Some colleagues may actually appreciate the little push toward healthier eating at work, although a few may enjoy the role of diet saboteur. But it's worth the effort to ask.

- Today, support systems are available 24/7 to anyone via the Internet. Give it a try. Lurk for a while (which means read the messages but don't necessarily respond to any or leave any of your own). Whatever you need, whatever question you have or problem you're facing, another person is probably coping with the same concern. Search until you find the online support that's just right for you.

the ten steps to a finally thin life

Here are some Web site suggestions:

3fatchicks.com	healthyexchanges.com
aolhealth.com	hungrygirl.com
buddyslim.com	ivillage.com
diet.com	lowcarb.ca
diet-blog.com	sparkpeople.com
diettalk.com	thedietchannel.com
everydayhealth.com	webmd.com
extrapounds.com	weightwatchers.com
health.msn.com	weightloss.about.com
health.yahoo.com	

• And of course, you've always got me: kimbensen.com.

you're not superman, but . . .

There will be times when you'll want that package of cookies so bad, you won't remember (for a moment, anyway) why it was so important to stick to your diet. What can you do to vanquish that urge?

Wouldn't it be great to *be* Superman? You wouldn't have to struggle to keep the house in shape, you'd be caught up at the office, and you'd have the kids in line in no time! You'd be physically fit, indestructible, tireless, strong, superfast.

Wait . . . did I say *indestructible*? But he wasn't. There was this little thing called kryptonite. When he was near it, he grew weaker and weaker. If he didn't escape or get rescued, he'd die from it. Well, he never *really* died. Someone always saved him, but he *could have* died. Remember?

Recently, at one of the weight loss meetings I lead, this notion came to mind as I was describing the strong force food can still exert over you. It

Whether you think you can, or whether you think you can't . . . you're right.
—*Henry Ford*

draws you in, makes you feel powerless, weakens you much as kryptonite weakens Superman.

And, like kryptonite, your proximity to the food directly impacts how much power it has over you. Just think about when you pass through the kitchen and a plate of something yummy is on the counter, looking oh-so-delicious. Your eyes go to it, you envision yourself cutting a slice, and you suddenly *really* want some. You try to put it out of your mind, but your thoughts keep returning to it. You remember its taste and texture, and you know how close it is. And so the desire to eat it grows.

It's the same with cleaning up leftovers. That meatloaf and mashed potatoes tasted way too good to let the pleasure end. You're handling them and wrapping them up—and you can't resist the urge to finish the last few ounces on your little one's plate. (I know I'm not the only one who has eaten my kid's leftovers!)

For people with overeating struggles, food can be just like kryptonite, bringing a strong woman to her knees and leaving her weak and frustrated. If nothing intervenes, it can mean death (well, the death of her diet).

Here's the important thing: The food becomes *powerless* when it's inside its lead box. (For you non-Superman buffs, kryptonite couldn't hurt Superman if it was behind lead. *Duh!*) Once the food is out of sight—put away, thrown out, or sent home with a guest—it loses all power to destroy.

Sometimes even Superman needed help to survive the kryptonite. As strong as he was, he wouldn't have made it without the help of Lois Lane or Jimmy Olson. The same is true for us, and we need to be willing to *ask* for that help.

Ask guests to take their unfinished dessert home with them. Insist!

Ask someone else to put leftovers away while you chat and load the dishwasher.

Ask your family to eat fewer fast-food meals out—and instead offer options for healthier choices.

Enlisting support and asking for help: two more baby steps to get you where you want to go.

exercise your
right to move

*When I weighed nearly 350 pounds, I couldn't walk around the
block, let alone manage a workout routine. When I got down to
around 250 pounds, I started thinking, "I have to do something to
tighten up all of this loose skin!" I got down on my hands and
knees and tried to do a girly push-up (knees bent). As I tried to
push myself back up, I fell flat on my face. I rolled over, defeated.
The next day, I tried again. The same result. For two weeks I was
unable to do a push-up. But then one day it happened. I did my
first girly push-up—woo-hoo! The next week it was three. Within
four months I was able to do twenty "guy" push-ups, and I have
been doing them ever since. My routine today—twenty guy push-
ups and a hundred crunches—takes only four minutes, but I
make sure it's the first thing I do every morning. I found what
works for me and have stuck with it for nearly five years now. Is it
the best program in the world? No. I'm still a work in progress.
Today I also work out at either Curves or Planet Fitness, trying to
make sure I get in that cardio that is so good for my body. But it
took me five years to work up to this level of commitment.*

Even I—a reluctant exerciser—appreciate the dozens of reasons for
making the time to get in shape. As you move closer and closer to
your goal weight, your body will require less and less food. One

way to be able to eat a little more is to move a little more! And exercise has many other benefits:

- Strengthens the cardiovascular and respiratory systems

- Reduces the risk of osteoporosis, keeping bones and muscles strong

- Prevents and manages type 2 diabetes

- Eases depression and stress

- Reduces risks of certain types of cancers

- Improves sleep, including reducing sleep disorders

- Helps manage weight loss and maintenance

- Promotes a longer, healthier life

Not only do you reap the immediate benefits of the calories you have burned, but exercise increases the body's metabolic rate. And that can be very important for long-term weight loss success.

getting started

If you and exercise mix like oil and water, join the club. We're not alone. They say that seven out of ten American adults don't exercise regularly, even with all the proven health benefits. That's a pretty large club.

Despite the fact that I lost 212 pounds, exercise played a fairly small part in my weight loss. This is good news if you want proof that you can lose a lot of weight even if you don't exercise. On the other hand, exercise is vitally important for better health.

The right kind of exercise can help you develop cardiovascular endurance, muscular strength, and flexibility. When you work out aerobically, more blood is pumped through your veins, which increases their size. This prevents fat from clogging your arteries, keeps blood clots from forming, lowers your blood pressure, increases good cholesterol, and lowers overall cholesterol. If that isn't persuasive enough, other benefits include stress relief and reduced risk of some chronic diseases, including diabetes and osteoporosis.

Wow! I need to get me some of that!

New government guidelines suggest that people, especially those with sedentary jobs, who get only thirty minutes per day of exercise are still likely to be at risk for weight gain and its complications. The new recommendations have doubled to an hour per day of moderate physical exercise—though vigorous exercise can cut that in half. The good news is, it's fine if you break exercise down into smaller sessions—say, walking your dog, taking the stairs at work, or getting off the bus a stop or two early.

Regular aerobic exercise will give you the most respiratory and cardio benefits, but any physical activity has value. If your main interest is fat loss, the experts recommend doing cardio every day, with a few days of strength training thrown in—works like magic. Whatever you choose, remember: The more you enjoy it, the more likely you will stick with it.

increased activity

Everything you do burns calories—including breathing, lying in bed, and wiggling your ears! Of course, they don't burn very many, but it's nice to know that no time is wasted. Working out every day is a great goal, but if formal exercise isn't part of your daily life right now, think about other sources of activity. All those little tips that you've always heard, such as parking farther away in a parking lot or taking the stairs instead of the elevator, really do make a difference. Here's a fun list to give you an idea of how many calories you can burn with everyday activities. The following burn calories equivalent to low-impact aerobics:

- Gardening

- Sailing

- Hunting

- Wallpapering

- Snorkeling

- Vigorous playing with your children—or someone else's

A person who weighs 155 pounds will burn 352 calories per hour performing any of these. The same individual doing one full hour of heavy house cleaning will burn 317 calories. Think of it—you can burn those calories and have a clean house too!

Here are five important steps to take before you start:

Step 1: Check with your doctor.

You don't want to get hurt before you get started. It's easy to push your body too hard the first time out—and then find yourself in so much pain you can't continue. Start slowly and keep increasing as your body adjusts.

Step 2: Choose the right fitness program.

You gotta love it or you won't do it! Try different things. If you don't like the gym setting at all, try some kind of dance, square dancing, karate, or zumba. Spend two weeks trying out all different sorts of alternative exercises. Pick the one you like best and make a short-term commitment, then reevaluate at the end.

Step 3: Set goals.

Setting goals helps you keep track of your progress. One of my goals was to be able to do a "guy push-up." I sure knew it when I reached that goal—and so did everyone else in the house. *Woo-hoo!* For *SIMPLE* goal-setting guidelines, check out page 93.

Step 4: Get going.

Just do it! Make sure you have everything you need to do what you've chosen. Consider breaking up your workouts if that's best or you. Health experts agree that you can get nearly the same benefit from three ten-minute walks as one thirty-minute walk. Even starting with a four-minutes-a-day routine is just that—a start. Remember, *some* routine is better than *none*.

Step 5: Track your progress.

When it's on paper, it's easier to see. Sometimes progress is so slow, you may not notice that you're getting stronger and more fit. Make sure you take your measurements before you begin and watch those inches decrease. Also notice other health improvements in areas such as energy, attitude, blood pressure, and cholesterol.

the ten steps to a finally thin life

Don't feel you have to pick one thing and do it forever. In fact, changing your workout several times a week—or several times a year—is a terrific idea. Keep it interesting, keep it challenging, and keep it going.

don't forget walking!

Experts agree that most people *over*estimate how much they move and *under*estimate how much they eat. Pedometers can keep us honest. Put one on when you get dressed each morning and see how many steps you've taken at the end of the day.

After supper check your pedometer. If you haven't reached your daily goal, go out and take a walk. Increase slowly each day until you have hit your target range.

important things to remember about walking

- Always check with your physician before beginning *any* exercise program.

- Walking may not always be easy, but it shouldn't hurt. If it does, get checked out.

- Breathing should not be too labored. If you are pushing yourself, your breathing will be elevated, but you should never be gasping. (Try the "Talk Test": Can you answer a question easily? You are walking too slowly. Can you not answer a question at all? You are walking too fast.)

- Stretch before and after walking to prevent injury.

step counting for healthy adults

Under 5,000 steps/day = sedentary

5,000 to 7,499 steps/day = low active

7,500 to 9,999 steps/day = somewhat active

10,000 steps/day = active

In the 1940s when secretaries switched from the old manual type-writers to the lighter-touch electric typewriters, it has been calculated that their energy expenditure was reduced by about 200 calories a day. Providing nothing else in their lives changed, that would mean a weight gain of twenty pounds in the course of one year. Small changes really do add up!

kinds of exercise

CARDIOVASCULAR—primarily benefits your heart, circulatory system, and lungs.

STRENGTH AND MUSCLE ENDURANCE—primarily benefits you by making you stronger and/or giving you better endurance, so you can do things longer.

FLEXIBILITY—primarily aimed at giving you greater range of motion in joints and more suppleness in your body.

Some other things to think about include the following:

INTENSITY (HOW HARD?)—Intensity can vary from very light to very hard and can be monitored on the basis of training heart rate or your own subjective impression of how hard you are working.

FREQUENCY (HOW MANY?)—Start with three days a week and work toward seven days a week.

DURATION (HOW LONG?)—Begin with a minimum of twenty minutes throughout a day with a goal of increasing to sixty minutes a day. This can be done in multiple fifteen-minute sessions or in one longer session.

A safe exercise routine consists of three parts:

WARM-UP: Five minutes of light activity, such as slow walking or cycling.

ACTIVITY: Cardiovascular, muscular strength, or flexibility training.

COOLDOWN: Five minutes of light activity with some flexibility exercises built in.

family fitness—an idea for more "together time"

Another great way to incorporate exercise into your life is to bring the family along. Here are some fun ideas for getting fit as a family.

The simplest way to add some fitness minutes to your day is to walk instead of ride, or to allow extra time for a fast-paced stroll before you get where you're going. One of these may work for you and your kids:

- Instead of rushing for the bus at the last minute, plan to be ready fifteen minutes early, and stride a couple of lengths of your block before the bus arrives. Make it fun by playing word games as you walk, or let your son or daughter teach you the lyrics to a favorite song. Can your daughter name all the state capitals? Can your son walk and spell at the same time?

- When the family hits the mall, plan to cover a quick lap of the level you enter on, then climb the stairs to the next level and do it again. You can check out the sales and plan your visit as you walk down each and every corridor. Skip the food court—those aromas can be *dangerous*!

- The family that rides together gets strong together! What better way to add fitness to your family life than to plan a bike ride around your neighborhood before or after dinner?

- Put on a CD and invite everybody to dance up a storm while dinner is bubbling away on the stove.

- Buy each child a pedometer (only a few dollars at most pharmacies) and see who takes the most steps each day. If dinnertime approaches and everyone needs a few more steps, get out there and power-walk!

- Want to up the ante? Suggest that the family enter an upcoming charity fund-raising walk and train together for it.

> When will you find time for exercise?
> After you have your first heart attack?
> —*Jean Bensen, my mother-in-law*

learn to eat light at home and away

In the summer of 1994, Mark and I took Aleeta and Adam on a weekend trip to beautiful Lancaster, Pennsylvania. It was during this trip that one of the most humiliating things ever happened to me, something so bad that I still cringe when I think about it.

Driving back to our hotel after touring a pretzel factory, we spotted a sign for Ed's Buggy Rides off the main street and pulled in. Ed was a soft-spoken farmer whose buggy had been in his family for generations—and it looked like his horse had, too. We chatted pleasantly with him about his family and Amish life in general. More than anything I wanted to take my family on an Amish buggy ride.

I stood next to Ed's buggy. Now I'm no engineer, but I just can't believe that the whole size thing never entered my mind. I was so consumed with the nostalgia, the romance of a buggy ride with my little family, clip-clopping our way through the picturesque countryside, that I never considered whether I would even fit in Ed's tired black buggy.

I don't know why Ed didn't say anything. He must have been able to size up the situation. Maybe he needed the money. Maybe he was too much of a gentleman. But Ed said nothing, and I was blissfully unaware of the pending problem until it was time to go. I eagerly stuck my head and shoulders through the opening. In one brief, horrible moment, hovering between being inside the buggy and outside where I belonged, I knew I would never fit.

It took me only a second to realize what I had not foreseen earlier. The inside sported a short bench directly behind the driver's seat and a full bench across the back of the buggy, not unlike a minivan today but on a much smaller scale. I wouldn't fit width-wise on the short bench, and both benches were too narrow for my derriere. Even if I did somehow make it into the buggy, there was just no suitable spot for me to sit.

The reality of my situation hit me like a physical blow. Everyone was behind me, waiting for me to get in. I backed out quickly and suggested that Mark and our excited kids get in first.

As my family bounded into the buggy, panic welled up in me. What was I going to do? I just wouldn't fit! It was Ed who came to my rescue, "Wait now a moment. We have a seat used usually by our mothers-in-law which you may find more comfortable." Comfortable! Hah! The dear man was trying to help. He pulled a small wooden block from the back of the buggy and placed it on the floor next to the short bench. This extended the back seat another foot or so in depth. It might just work. I wouldn't know until I tried it. Now to get in.

Mark was already in the corner of the rear bench. Adam and Aleeta were seated on the short bench in the middle. I put my foot up on the buggy and pulled myself up onto the edge of the doorway, twisting as best I could to the right. Mark and the kids pulled from the inside, which I don't think helped any, but one purposeful shove on my derriere by Ed's shoulder from the outside and I finally popped into the buggy. I twisted more around as I fell and plopped ungracefully down onto the mother-in-law stool. I was in!

I thought the buggy was going to tip over. Ed's horse startled and neighed. Ed scrambled up onto his seat and we were off.

Ed was both entertaining and informative during our half-hour trip through town and countryside, but the entire time all I could think of was, "How am I ever going to get out of here?" I was blocking the exit for everyone else as well. I could imagine the headlines: "FAMILY TRAPPED IN ED'S BUGGY—JAWS OF LIFE NEEDED TO FREE THEM."

Just when I thought nothing worse could happen, the buggy went over a bump just big enough to give us all a jolt, just enough for me to put a little more pressure on my already overburdened seat, just enough for me to break it!

I felt and heard the wood crack and began listing decidedly to the left. Poor Ed. Poor Ed's mother-in-law. Poor me! I wanted to scream in frustration. I wanted to hide in humiliation. How was I ever going to tell him? I thought for sure Ed would think he had a flat tire—or a busted spoke or something. But amazingly no one else had heard. The tour went on uninterrupted.

We were soon pulling back into Ed's driveway. Getting out was worse than I had imagined. I just couldn't fit unless I was sideways, and that was a very difficult position to maneuver at my size and in the cramped amount of space—and on a broken stool! Having performed a similar feat just a half hour earlier, I began my comedic contortionist's routine and ultimately worked my way out of the buggy, breathing a sigh of relief when my feet hit the ground.

To my shame I didn't tell Ed about his busted stool. I was too humiliated to say anything to anyone, including Mark. We thanked Ed and I hustled everyone back to our car as quickly as I could, but for the rest of the weekend I watched over my shoulder for an irate Amish farmer. One of my goals in life is to eventually find Ed, apologize, and offer to pay for breaking his mother-in-law's stool.

lighten up at home

There are three basic ways you can eat fewer calories. You can:

1. Eat *less* of your current foods and recipes the way they're written (often, a lot less).

2. Lighten up your current foods and recipes by swapping out ingredients.

3. Find and try *new* lighter foods and recipes.

All three ways work, and one is not necessarily better than any other. I actually do a mixture of all three, and I bet most people will as well. But for me, the second and third methods are the ones that have made the difference—the ones that helped me finally get to goal and stay there.

I found that controlling my own recipes and using lower-fat ingredients enabled me to make and eat a higher volume of food, which kept

> Don't trade what you want most for
> what you want at the moment.

me satisfied. More food, fewer calories, more taste, less fat! At 350 pounds, that's exactly what I needed. I could whip up a stir-fry that would rival anything high-fat that I'd ever made before—and at a fraction of the calories. To me, that meant I didn't have to eat small portions and feel hungry. I could satisfy my urge to eat and chew and still continue to lose.

Today I *desire* to eat less than I used to because my body is smaller and my habits have changed. But that change came slowly, over quite a long time. In the beginning my goal was to eat enough great-tasting food that I felt full and satisfied and enjoyed what I was doing. This bought me the time I needed to work on those small behavioral changes along the way.

what do you really know about portion sizes?

With the onslaught of supersized meals came the onslaught of the supersized waistline. Americans' view of proper portion sizes has become distorted, and it's not just at the drive-through. We're surrounded by larger portion sizes at relatively low prices, which appeals to our pocketbooks. The problem is, you do pay more for it—in clogged arteries, overburdened hearts, high blood pressure, and ultimately, in serious health problems.

The U.S. Department of Health and Human Services has a great quiz you can take online that compares serving sizes twenty years ago to those we are offered today. Visit my Web site (kimbensen.com) for a direct link.

Here are two examples from it:

- Twenty years ago the adult cheeseburger order was just that . . . a cheeseburger (333 calories). Today, you can order from a double cheeseburger to a quadruple cheeseburger. The total: from 550 to more than 1,000 calories.

- An average popcorn used to be 5 cups, for a total of 270 calories. Today, 630 calories is considered a medium-sized portion (without the extra butter), and many moviegoers consume lots more.

Remember, there's a difference between *serving size* and *portion size.* Statistics show that if someone is given a larger portion of food, even if it's the equivalent of two servings, they'll eat it. For example, most people don't realize that a serving size for potato chips is 1 ounce; instead, we gobble down the contents of a 2½ ounce (small) bag. The print is small, the chips are tasty—how easy it is to ignore the fact that you're eating more than 300 calories instead of 170.

Our bodies really need very little food to grow and be healthy, compared to how much we like to eat. Sad, isn't it? The sooner we realize what a modest number of calories we need, the sooner we can get our diets into perspective. Instead of succumbing to the distorted realities of what we see on television and in print ads, on billboards and menus, we need to get real about the number of calories our bodies needs to function. And it ain't much!

is any food really free?

FREE FOOD! No, I'm not talking cost. It's a term used by many diets to identify foods that are allowed on a relatively unlimited basis. Celery is usually on the list. Depending on what program you follow, it could mean an array of nonstarchy vegetables or it may mean a food item that has little to no net carbs. One thing is for certain: chocolate cake is *not* on the list.

Whatever "free food" means to you, these food items can be consumed in quantity and frequency to fill the gaping void left behind as we give up unlimited eating and try to follow a diet regimen. And I was grateful for every item on my list!

One question I am frequently asked is, "Is it possible to gain weight on 'free foods'?" My answer is yes. No food item has zero calories. Eaten in large quantities, the caloric amount of these "free foods" does add up.

So although you *can* eat larger quantities of these "free foods" for less, the quantity you consume still has to be considered. Many of us with

We used to go to a Mexican restaurant that offered free tortilla chips and salsa. I started bringing a bag of baby carrots in my purse to dip in the salsa. It was great! So great, in fact, that everyone else joined in my carrot idea. One bag doesn't stretch far, but I soon learned to bring more.

weight problems keep eating past the point of fullness not because we are hungry, but because we like eating. And we have a hard time recognizing when we are full.

Use your "free foods"—just don't ab*use* them. You will likely pay for it in other ways as well, such as cramping and gas.

visualize your portion size

These are some great visual aids to help you get a clear mental picture of what a serving looks like—and what a real portion should be:

- 4 dice or 1 Matchbox car = 1 ounce (cheese)

- Ping-Pong ball = 2 tablespoons (peanut butter or salad dressing)

- golf ball = 4 tablespoons or ¼ cup (raisins or nuts)

- deck of cards = 3 ounces (sliced meat)

- tennis ball = 1 ounce (cereal) or ½ cup (ice cream)

My favorite portion control helper is just using my hands. The palm of your hand is about 3 ounces. Clench your fist to visualize 8 fluid ounces. The tip of your thumb is 1 teaspoon and two thumbs equals 1 tablespoon. Cupping both your hands together is approximately equal to 1 cup, and one hand cupped is a half a cup. These are approximations, of course, and vary according to the size of your hands, but it's a good rule of thumb (pun intended) when you have nothing else to help you measure your food.

In most cases, eating smaller portions really helps cut back on calories. If you're like me and prefer a fuller plate, you'll need to "pile on" larger quantities of lower-calorie foods such as vegetables.

Here's a great visual for you. Hold both your fists out together in front of you. Go on, do it. Okay, take a good look. That's about the size of your stomach. If you are eating more food than that, your stomach is going to start expanding and you will be eating beyond full. Look again. It *isn't* a lot of food!

water, water everywhere

Seventy percent—that's the number to remember. Water makes up 70 percent of your body, so it's pretty important to keep your body well hydrated. Most diet plans suggest a minimum of six to eight glasses of water per day; others use a formula based on body weight.

I have to work at drinking my water. I'm not a natural water lover, though I envy those who are. I'd rather drink Diet Coke, much to my mother's chagrin. My mom likes to send me e-mails about the benefits of water and the many reasons to avoid my carbonated "poison" of choice. And although there are plenty of days when I fall short of my targeted water consumption, I keep those good reasons in mind as I try to make better beverage choices.

my mom's favorite reasons to drink your water

1. You can live for a month without food (really!) but only about a week without water. It's vital to survival.

2. Water helps with weight loss (really!), as it increases your metabolism and regulates your appetite. Did you know that we often mistake thirst for hunger? (I mistake a *lot* of things for hunger, but quenching my thirst is an easy fix.)

3. Water has other health benefits, including reducing the risk of certain types of cancer, such as colon, bladder, and breast cancers. It aids circulation, as it transports nutrients throughout the body and flushes out waste and bacteria that can cause disease.

4. It's a wonderful beauty treatment—not just *on* your skin but *in* it! Improving hydration in your skin cells causes them to plump up nicely when they might otherwise sag due to aging or weight loss. *I gotta get me some of that!*

I'm sure there may be other reasons, but aren't survival, weight loss, better health, and beauty a pretty good start? But how do you know how much to drink? Forty-eight ounces—the typical six glasses of 8 ounces each—are not always the ideal target.

Some researchers believe that for every twenty-five pounds of excess weight you carry, you should add another 8-ounce glass. But that's a lot of water. When I weighed 350 pounds, by that measure, I should have been drinking more than 112 ounces of water every day. Yowza!

Other factors to consider are the following:

YOUR ACTIVITY LEVEL—You'll want to drink additional water before and during sweaty workouts. As your body loses water, it needs to be replaced, *before* you feel thirsty. Once you feel your thirst, your body is already beginning to experience dehydration.

THE CLIMATE IN WHICH YOU LIVE—If you perspire more than usual in a tropical setting or during a heat wave, make sure you keep drinking steadily through the day.

HOW MUCH FLUID YOU LOSE BY DRINKING CAFFEINE (A DIURETIC), DURING NURSING, OR BECAUSE OF SICKNESS SUCH AS DIARRHEA—It's a good idea to switch to noncaffeinated sodas if you drink them regularly.

A cool online water calculator can help you figure out the right amount of water for *you*. There's a link on my Web site (kimbensen. com). I took the quiz recently, and here's what it told me:

A person who is 135 pounds and is exercising for 30 minutes daily, is not pregnant, is not breastfeeding, does not live at a high altitude, does not live in a dry climate, drinks 0 alcoholic drink(s), when the weather is not very hot or very cold, and is not sick with fever or diarrhea should have:

70.5 ounces of water today.

If you eat a healthy diet, about 20 percent of your water may come from the foods you eat. If you eat a healthy diet you can drink 56.4 ounces of water today.

That's what it told me. Pretty neat, don't you think? A few more things to remember about water:

- You don't have to drink it all at once.

- You can add nondiuretic flavorings to the water—Crystal Light, decaf coffee, and herbal teas, for instance (watch for added calories).

- Seltzer counts. Add a squeeze and a slice of fresh lime or lemon.

- Ice counts! Shaved ice is *great* with a little sugar-free syrup—a homemade snow cone.

- It doesn't matter when you drink your water during the day, but it's a *really* good idea to stop drinking three hours before bedtime. You know why.

If drinking water has always been one of the areas you struggled with while dieting, think of it this way: There are a lot of things we *should* do to keep our bodies healthy that are pretty difficult—increasing activity, decreasing portion sizes, not eating food items that we sometimes crave. Drinking more water is not all that difficult, and the benefits are huge.

Thanks, Mom, you were right!

lighten up away from home

When we cook meals at home, we can figure out what's in the food we prepare using calorie guides, points finders, and the ever-present nutrition label. But when we go out to eat, we're at the mercy of the restaurant, the fast-food joint, and the takeout counter. The most critical thing I have to tell you is—*know before you go.* Don't put it in your mouth unless you know what's in it. Surveys show that most people don't have any idea of the food values for what they eat outside the home. Until I started doing research, I never imagined how far off I could be in assuming something was healthy when it was not.

That's another good piece of advice: *Never assume anything when eating out.* Don't tell yourself that if it's on the salad bar, it's healthy. Don't feel certain that if it says *sugar-free* or has a heart-smart symbol, it's low in calories. Don't assume *anything.* If you don't know what's in it, don't eat it until you do.

When I became the diet editor for Better TV, I began traveling into New York City each week to film a "Lighten Up! with Kim Bensen" segment. One of my favorites is when we play "Dare to Compare." I set out several pairs of food items and asked Audra, one of the show's hosts, to pick which ones she thinks have less fat and fewer calories. She is frequently mistaken. There are more hidden calories than we realize!

Here are three "Know Before You Go" examples:

McDonald's	vs.	Costco
Large Fries		Double Chocolate Chip Muffin
570 calories, 30 g fat		**690 calories, 38 g fat**

McDonald's	vs.	Dunkin' Donuts
Quarter Pounder		Wheat Bagel with Cream Cheese
420 calories, 18 g fat		**520 calories, 21 g fat**

Burger King	vs.	Chili's
Double Whopper with Cheese		Shrimp Caesar Salad
890 calories, 50 g fat		**980 calories, 77 g fat**

Surprised? That's the point. How many times have you said, "Oh, I'll only have a muffin for breakfast"? It doesn't seem like much, does it? And what about that wheat bagel with cream cheese? The light cream cheese version, by the way, still has more fat and calories than the Quarter Pounder. And that's for only 2 ounces of cream cheese, not the 4 ounces they often smear on.

tips for healthy dining

Here are some healthy dining tips to help you reduce the volume of food you consume at restaurants and at home.

Eating Out

1. Plan to split an entrée with another person.

2. Ask your server to wrap up part of your meal before he or she even brings it to the table.

3. Order an appetizer or side dish for an entrée.

4. Order from the lunch menu at dinnertime. (They don't advertise this option, but it often exists.)

5. You *don't* want to supersize, thank you. You may get the question, so have the answer ready!

6. Kids' meals are a better choice at fast-food restaurants. Why? They are a more appropriate serving size for an adult.

7. Don't be afraid to special-order. Ask for substitutions, speak up, and get what you need. You're paying for it, after all.

8. Order sauces and dressings on the side. This way you choose how much to use. When eating your salad, dip your fork into the dressing first and then grab a forkful of salad. You'll get just the right amount of dressing for that mouthful!

9. Be careful of restaurant-made, tomato-based sauces (they can have lots of added oil) and light dressings (some are lighter than others).

10. Ask for foods grilled, broiled, steamed, baked, dry-sautéed, or poached—but make it clear that you do not want any added butters or oils.

11. Say no to fried foods, gravies, cheese toppings, and cream-based sauces and soups. (Broccoli cheese soups are not a good way to get your veggies!)

12. Make sure meats are lean and skinless. If the dish comes with the skin, just peel it off and set it to the side. Trim excess fat. Round is the lightest cut of meat; ribs are the heaviest.

At Home

13. Plate your meals in the kitchen at home and keep serving dishes off the table at mealtimes.

14. Use lunch plates instead of dinner plates, especially when serving yourself.

15. Go for whole grains whenever possible.

16. Minimize processed foods. You'll eat a lot less sodium.

17. Limit sugary sodas and other high-calorie beverages. Remember, a tall glass of orange juice contains nearly 200 calories! Think of soda as liquid candy bars.

18. Do use mustards, vinegars, herbs, salsas, and fat-free dressings.

19. Keep foods in opaque containers so they don't tempt you when you open the fridge or cabinets. Label them instead.

20. Keep your kitchen stocked with healthy foods. If getting to the store is difficult, consider using an online delivery service such as Peapod or Fresh Direct.

the ten steps to a finally thin life

Here's another example of how even someone with lots of experience making healthy choices can blow it. I went to our local Ruby Tuesday for dinner not long ago. I love their salad bar and eat there frequently. This particular evening, I wanted to have their petit sirloin steak to go with my salad bar, but as I glanced down the menu I decided instead to "be good" and ordered the veggie burger. *Big mistake!* When I got home, I looked up both items online and found that while the petit sirloin would have had 205 calories and 5 grams of fat, the veggie burger had nearly 1,000 calories and 46 grams of fat!

I blew it. I could have had *four* petit sirloin steaks and still have come out lower in fat and calories. See what happens when you're trying to be good—without being informed as well?

You have to know before you go. It's not as hard as it sounds. As long as you have access to the Internet, you can find out most of what you need to know. Simply type the restaurant's name and then the words *nutritional information* into any search engine and hit "go." You'll likely get a list of Web sites to visit. If the restaurant you're researching is there, click on it—that will be your most accurate source of information. But if it's not there, your search engine will give you some other options—sites that have figured out the fat, calories, carbs, and other data for that business's menu items. There is a link to the nutritional information for all the major fast-food joints and chains on kimbensen.com as well.

If you don't have access to the Web or you can't find what you need to know, call ahead and ask if nutritional information is available. Chain restaurants typically provide it; individual establishments may not.

Knowing what your choices are ahead of time will help you make good choices *before* you are faced with the delicious sights and smells at the restaurant. If you can't get any information and you don't have a choice about the restaurant, it's smart to stick with basic foods such as steak, plain baked potato, grilled chicken, and salads with the dressing on the side. Ask to have your food prepared without added oils or butters.

A moment on the lips, a long time on the hips.

green-light restaurant terms

Baked	Fresh	Roasted
Boiled	Grilled	Steamed
Broiled	High fiber	
Fat free	Poached	

yellow-light restaurant terms

Crunchy	Multigrain	Stewed
Lite or light	Platter	Stir-fried
Marinated	Reduced	Vinaigrette

red-light restaurant terms

Au gratin	Cheesy	King size
Basted	Country-style	Loaded
Battered	Covered	Sauce (white or brown)
Béarnaise	Cream (creamed,	Sautéed
Bottomless	cream-style)	Smothered
Braised	Crispy	Stuffed
Breaded	Fried/deep fried	Supersized
Buttery/buttered	Giant	Value
Casserole	Gravy	

what about the salad bar?

Most dieters head straight for the salad bar if the restaurant has one. You figure, it's perfect to help you stay on your diet, right? *Not* necessarily! A plate of unwise salad bar choices can top out at 1,500 calories and 45 grams of fat! That's more than a Big Mac, fries, and a shake! *Yikes!*

Here are some few tips to make your next visit to the salad bar one that won't sabotage your healthy eating plan:

- *Guard against the "get your money's worth" mentality.* Anything all-you-can-eat is an invitation to excess.

- *Be adventurous.* Try a veggie or two that you've never tried before. This way, if you don't really love it, you haven't wasted your money buying an entire bunch or package.

- *Choose a fat-free dressing, salsa, or flavored vinegar.* The wrong dressing can turn a healthy salad into a very *unhealthy* one. Regular dressings can contain up to 180 calories and 20 grams of fat per serving (2 tablespoons), but it's the "low-fat" dressings that worry me. Lower than what? If the restaurant lists a dressing as "light," that simply means less than the original; they can still be loaded with calories. Fat-free dressings, salsas, and vinegars are your safest bet. Better yet—bring your own! (Here's my *Finally Thin* rule of thumb: Use only 1 tablespoon of light dressing; use 2 tablespoons of fat free. One full ladle is usually 2 tablespoons.)

- *Use the salad bar as a handy takeout option.* Those precut veggies can be a convenient quick start for homemade soups and stir-fries. Buying them from a salad bar can save prep time. And that means time away from the kitchen.

Use my helpful charts (see pages 146–147) to plan your next visit to the salad bar.

drive-through dieting

Twenty years ago the average American family went out to eat once a month. Today if you don't eat out several times a week, you are in the minority. It's not that I recommend eating on the run, but the fact is it's part of our lives. And because fast-food restaurants have become a major meal provider in the American lifestyle, with the drive-through or the corner booth replacing the family table for many meals during the week, the worst thing we can do is ignore it. Drive-through dieting is possible. I admit it. I do it several nights each week, and I manage to stay within my recommended healthy guidelines and calorie range at the same time. But it takes effort and education. I love to eat out. If I had to give that up, I probably would not have stuck with my diet. But instead I worked it all into my plan, including the once deadly fast food.

Hard to believe? It's true. I eat at McDonald's several times a week. I usually get their Grilled Asian Chicken Salad. It's loaded with mixed greens, snow peas, mandarin oranges, red peppers, and edamame. If I skip the packet of almonds and use one-third of the packet of dressing, it's only 280 calories. Not a bad lunch for fast food on the go, right? And I top it off with a vanilla cone—only 150 calories (as long as they give me no more than three swirls). How do I know? I asked a manager.

Enjoy!

Let's face it . . . going on vacation often means vacationing from our weight-loss regimen as well. We work so hard to look good for vacation. But many of us, with our all-or-nothing personalities, find it hard to indulge "just a little," and when we fall, we fall *big-time*! The even bigger problem can be getting back on track when the vacation is over.

One way to avoid this trap is to make weight goals for vacation.

1. Are you going strong and want to keep losing on this vacation? Great! Pack a cooler and take the products you need with you. Call ahead to where you're going and fit in some special meals while still keeping the calories low. Plan and prepare!

2. Don't want to gain on vacation, but aren't too concerned about losing either? Great! Plan on increasing your caloric intake a little (even more if you add some extra activity into each day). Keeping your diet on a maintenance level can give you some extras you want to have without a gain in the end.

3. Don't want to think about your diet this vacation? Great! If this is your plan, feel free to treat yourself, making sure you don't lose control. Have dessert each night; just don't have ten desserts! Enjoy one special, relaxing, three-hour, seven-course meal; just don't do it three meals a day for the entire vacation.

Whatever you do, do it in control. And most important, no matter what happens on vacation, make a plan to get back to your meeting, to your trainer, to your support group, on your food plan . . . the moment you return!

Get informed before you go. I always say, the fewer surprises the better. Check out the nutritional information for restaurants and fast-food joints that you may be visiting. Call your cruise line or facility ahead of time to find out what special menus may be available to you. This is not unusual, nor is it rude. It's getting what you need. It's taking care of yourself, and it's an important part of getting ready for your vacation.

the ten steps to a finally thin life

salad bar nutrition information

Item	Portion	Calories	Fat (gm)	Total Carb (gm)	Sod (mg)	Fiber (gm)
artichoke hearts	½ cup	42	0	9.4	80	4.5
beets	½ cup	40	0	8	260	1
black olives	2 tbsp	30	2.5	0.1	140	0
broccoli florets	1 cup	31	0	6	30	2
carrots	½ cup	22	0	5.5	38	1.5
cauliflowerettes	1 cup	25	0	5.3	30	2.5
celery	½ cup	8	0	0	48	1
cucumbers	½ cup	8	0	2	1	0.5
lettuce	1 cup	8	0	2	6	1
mushrooms	1 cup	15	0	2.3	3.5	<1
onions	5 rings	12	0	3	1	<1
peas	⅔ cup	60	0	11	120	4
green peppers	½ cup	12	0	3.5	2.2	1
sweet peppers	½ cup	20	0.5	1	480	1
radishes	½ cup	10	0	2	23	<1
spinach	1 cup	7	0	1	24	<1
tomatoes	1 cup	32	0	7	9	2

Miscellaneous Toppers

Item	Portion	Calories	Fat (gm)	Total Carb (gm)	Sod (mg)	Fiber (gm)
bacon bits	¼ cup	98	7	0	880	0
beans (kidney, garbanzo, etc.)	¼ cup	56	0.5	9.5	222	2
Cheddar cheese	1 oz	114	9.4	<1	176	0
chickpeas	½ cup	110	1	17	180	3.5
chow mein noodles, fried	½ cup	118	7	12.5	87	1
croutons	⅛ cup	66	2.6	9	176	<1
eggs	each	70	4	0	55	0
ham, cubed	2 oz	110	9	2	760	0
potato sticks	½ cup	94	6.2	9.6	45	0.6
raisins	2 tbsp	42	0	11	2	0.5
sunflower seeds	2 tbsp	110	9	1.2	60	2

NOTE: While these nutritional values are an excellent guide, they are approximations taken from an average of many government and commercial sources. Actual numbers will vary. Check online or call ahead to get more accurate nutritional information from the restaurant of your choice.

www.kimbensen.com

finally thin!

Prepared Salads and Sides

Item	Portion	Calories	Fat (gm)	Total Carb (gm)	Sod (mg)	Fiber (gm)
broccoli salad	4 oz	70	3	8	150	3
coleslaw	½ cup	160	10.3	17	434	<1
cottage cheese	½ cup	116	5	3	458	0
fruit, melon	¼ cup	15	0	3.6	6	<1
fruit, pineapple	¼ cup	19	0	5	<1	0.5
fruit, strawberries	¼ cup	13	0	3.2	0.7	0.8
fruit salad	⅓ cup	50	0	11	130	1
grilled chicken strips	4 oz	140	3	3	120	<1
macaroni salad	½ cup	216	11	26	480	1
potato salad	½ cup	190	10	24	576	1.5
three bean salad	⅓ cup	50	0	11	130	1
tuna salad	¼ cup	96	5	5	206	0
Waldorf salad	½ cup	160	2	38	0	3

Salad Dressings

Item	Portion	Calories	Fat (gm)	Total Carb (gm)	Sod (mg)	Fiber (gm)
balsamic vinaigrette	2 tbsp	60	5	4	190	0
blue cheese dressing	2 tbsp	170	18.5	1.5	309	0
Caesar dressing	2 tbsp	150	16	1	302	0
fat-free Italian dressing	2 tbsp	15	0	2	316	0
fat-free ranch dressing	2 tbsp	30	0	7	290	0
French dressing	2 tbsp	140	13	5	260	0
Italian dressing	2 tbsp	91	8	3	463	0
1000 island dressing	2 tbsp	150	15	5	274	0
lite Caesar dressing	2 tbsp	78	6	3	280	0
lite Italian dressing	2 tbsp	56	6	2	398	0
lite ranch dressing	2 tbsp	80	6	5	260	0
ranch dressing	2 tbsp	148	16	1	287	0
oil & vinegar (50/50)	2 tbsp	138	14	<1	0	0
vinegar	2 tbsp	8	0	1.8	0	0

learn to handle temptation

Journal entry: April 2000

I drove through Huntington Center today. As I approached the town green, the thought came to me, "I could just stop at the bakery and get an assortment of goodies to eat." But I was doing so well on my diet—I was determined not to blow it!

Traffic slowed, and I glanced over at the bakery window dressed in white wedding cakes. They made some of the best cake I had ever tasted. I wondered if they were crowded. I decided to peek and see. I needed rolls for dinner anyway. I pulled into the parking lot and looked in the window.

No long line. Well, I could go in and just get the rolls and leave. I knew I had to hurry because I still had to stop at my local grocery store for a few other items before starting supper. I should just get the rolls there and bypass the bakery, but . . . I was already here. I ran in quickly and headed to the counter. Inside the store the succulent odors assailed me. I glanced over at some of my old favorites. NO! I wouldn't! What was I doing here? This was too hard! There were the frosted brownies waiting as always. I knew they had granulated sugar on the bottom, a pleasant surprise the first time I had one. And today they had bear claws—usually sold out. And, oh! I loved those . . . it was my turn.

"Yes. I'd like. I'd like. Ummmmm. A dozen dinner rolls. And, uh, two of those frosted brownies and . . ."

had lost again. The battle lasted less than seven minutes.

But where did I lose the battle?

When I ate everything on my ride home? *No.* It was when I first thought, "I could just stop at the bakery—"

That was the crucial moment. When a thought first pops into our minds, it's so *little* then! We can handle that and get rid of it without much pain at all. But even that tiny thought feels good for a moment. We don't want to let it go too quickly. We want to stroke it, remember, touch, and taste in our minds. We often don't recognize it for the destructive force that it is. For whatever reason, we allow our minds to continue down the path of destruction when we could have saved ourselves so much pain. And if we don't *immediately* say a resounding NO! and change the direction of our thoughts before they have a chance to take hold of us, then we have picked up the gauntlet and the battle has begun.

This does not mean that all is lost. Victories have certainly been won at many points in battle, even when all seemed lost. I have on several occasions pitched the fattening goody I was eating *after* purchasing it. But it was very painful, not to mention costly, and I wished I had spared myself the emotional and financial expense.

How do we keep our eyes on the real goal, the big picture, the dream?

Where do we find the strength and the courage to break with past behaviors, to drive down a different street so we're not tempted by a bakery?

It's not really about hunger most of the time anyway. It's appetite, a learned response to a delicious aroma. You've probably heard at some point, "Oh, you're not *really* hungry. That's just *head* hunger!"

What do they mean, *just* head hunger? Of course it's head hunger—that terrible craving deep inside even when there are no physical signs of hunger.

I didn't get to weigh 350 pounds because I was physically hungry. Head hunger is what really hurts!

Here's an analogy that I just love. Think of your mind as an empty room. (For some of us, that's a lot easier than for others.) When the thought or desire to eat something that's not part of your plan occurs, it is as though someone has tossed a ball into the room.

Stressed is *desserts* spelled backward.

The question is, *What are you going to do with that ball?* Are you going to play with it? Toss it around? Stroke it? Or are you going to throw it back out of the room? Someone determined to stick to the plan grabs the ball every single time the ball is tossed in—and throws it back out again as quickly as possible.

It doesn't matter how many times it gets thrown back.

Anything can trigger a thought of food—a scent, a TV commercial, a place, even a person. You can't control how often such a thought occurs, how often the ball is tossed to you, but you *do* have control over what you do with it.

Grab it fast! Throw it out! Say a resounding "No!" and turn your mind immediately to something else.

This is one thing I practiced over and over again, and it finally worked! It got easier and easier, and once I figured it out, I rarely ever again experienced that pain.

Remember how crucial those first few moments of desire can be. If you avoid the battle, you will win the war.

the pain of having two loves

That brings me to *ambivalence.* I always thought that when you were ambivalent toward something, it meant that you didn't care about it, that you could take it or leave it. The dictionary defines ambivalence as "uncertainty caused by the inability to make a choice; a simultaneous desire to do two opposite or conflicting things."

Isn't that exactly how it is in weight loss? You *know* you want to lose weight more than anything . . . except for those times when you feel you want to eat something even more. Ambivalence! So what do you do?

why struggle makes us stronger

In the early 1990s, an enclosed ecological system named Biosphere II was constructed in Oracle, Arizona, to explore the complex interactions within life systems. The trees inside the 3.15-acre structure quickly grew lush and beautiful, but then a strange thing happened. Without the wind to buffet them and strengthen the wood of their trunks, they grew weak. They began breaking, unable to support their own weight. In the end, their perfect environment became their downfall.

As much as we don't like to be faced with it, temptation is not a bad thing. It is a chance to recommit to your dream, a chance to say no and grow stronger as much as it is a chance to give in and blow it. The more you say no when you are tempted, the stronger you will grow and the easier it will get. Practice makes it golden!

So the next time you face temptation, recognize it as an opportunity. *Success breeds success.*

how can you tell whether your hunger is real?

Learning how to differentiate between physical hunger and emotional "head" hunger is a skill you need to develop. Both fill you with a strong desire to eat, but don't be fooled. Head hunger is much stronger than physical hunger. Discovering which is driving your desire means that *you* are in the driver's seat, not your stomach.

If you are physically hungry, only one thing will make the hunger disappear, and that is food. If, however, you realize that you are *not physically hungry* but still have the desire to eat, other activities may well satisfy your "hunger" without the unwanted side effects of excess fat and ill health.

What are the signs of hunger?

signs of head hunger	signs of physical hunger
• Comes on quickly, suddenly; you realize how much you want to eat	• Comes on gradually, intensifies as caloric tank gets depleted
• No physical signs (though we desperately search for them—was that a stomach growl or just gas?)	• Physical signs include stomach growling, gnawing, empty feeling that may escalate to light-headedness and lack of energy
• Strong, intense urge	• Would like to eat but not desperate, patient
• Often paired with strong emotions	• Not emotionally linked

signs of head hunger	signs of physical hunger
• Often involves desire or craving for a specific food	• Desire is for food, not necessarily one particular kind
• Unable to recognize fullness easily	• Stop when physically full

Be honest. Without honesty, none of this will work. If you know you are not physically hungry, but want to eat anyway, that's okay. *But* recognize it honestly and say so to yourself. If you can do this, you've taken a giant leap toward change. If you're not physically hungry, ask yourself: what am I *really* feeling? Here's a list for you to run through:

Angry	Fearful	Lovesick
Anxious	Frustrated	Overburdened
Bitter	Grateful	Paranoid
Bored	Grief-stricken	Relieved
Content	Guilty	Sad
Depressed	Happy	Stressed (*desserts* spelled backward)
Disappointed	Homesick	Tired
Discouraged	Inadequate	Wanting to procrastinate
Envious	Jealous	Worried
Excited	Lonely	Yearning

See how many other things you may be feeling besides hunger? These are all emotional triggers that send you in search of food.

I often think about eating when I am bored . . . or happy, lonely, stressed, relieved, and just wanting to procrastinate. Because I know that, I'm almost never without things to do, but when I have downtime and don't want to tackle the next e-mail or project or writing assignment, I catch myself thinking, "Hmm. What's to eat?!"

The next time you are feeling as if you *desperately* want to eat, stop and evaluate whether it's head or physical hunger, and then determine what's going on at the moment.

Do I really want to eat or is something eating me?

Having a mantra that you love to say to yourself when you are faced with temptation can be very helpful. I've had many people e-mail me that they love my saying, "The only way you'll never lose weight is if you stop trying."

One saying I used when, as a waitress, I was trying not to eat Bertucci's fabulous hot rolls was, "Nothing tastes as good as thin feels." But I also memorized some Bible verses that were a source of strength and encouragement to me. I'll share a few of my favorites with you:

> In my anguish I cried to the Lord and He answered by setting me free.—Psalm 118:5

> God is faithful. He will not let you be tempted more than you can handle, but will with the temptation also give you a way out.
> —1 Corinthians 10:13

> Praise the Lord . . . who satisfies your desires with good things.—Psalm 103:5

> Commit to the Lord whatever you do and your plans will be successful.—Proverbs 16:3

getting busy

Emotions are unavoidable, and food can and does sometimes serve as a pacifier for them. But that's not the only way to handle them. Finding what satisfies the urge to eat instead of food is going to be key in your weight loss.

One way to combat head hunger is to occupy yourself with something you like to do. You want to choose something that satisfies you emotionally, just as food might. The right activity can fill you up inside and distract you from thinking about food, keep you from peeking into cabinets and digging around the back of the fridge in hopes of finding a tasty tidbit.

But what should you do? This is the time to do an inventory of things you enjoy but often don't make time to do. I bet there are some you haven't thought of in ages that could do the trick. You need to take the time to figure out what may work for you—and make sure you have the materials on hand if the activity requires them. Here are some ideas:

WRITE Start keeping a journal; write a letter to the editor or a faraway friend.

WALK Choose a nearby neighborhood to explore; find a local walking trail or park.

CROCHET OR KNIT I love this for nighttime head hunger when you're normally decompressing in front of the TV. It keeps your hands busy and your mind occupied.

SCRAPBOOK Create albums for all your photographs and vacation mementos; start a weight loss album to chronicle your journey.

READ Join a book club. I love to head up to bed early with a hot cup of tea and read until I fall asleep. It really helps break my nighttime habits.

PLAY THE PIANO Make the time to practice and finally get good; learn a challenging piece and perform for family and friends.

CALL A FRIEND If you've got unlimited minutes, *use* them to stay in touch with people you don't see often but miss a lot.

COOK Instead of just watching the Food Network, print out some recipes and see if you can give Bobby Flay a run for his money— lightened up, of course.

E-MAIL Catch up with family and friends.

JOIN A CHAT ROOM Hop on when you're feeling hungry or needing support. It will get your mind off food and remotivate you at the same time.

CREATE YOUR OWN WEB PAGE They're free, easy, and fun! Search Google for *free web pages* and check them out.

PLAY A GAME OF TETRIS Improve your hand-eye coordination and show your kids you're still pretty cool.

WATCH A QUICK VIDEO ONLINE If you missed an episode of your favorite series, you're in luck—you can probably catch it on the Web!

WINDOW-SHOP Think of what you'd like to wear if you could wear *anything*, or buy for your house if you came into an inheritance; there's no charge for dreaming!

REORGANIZE When I have a few minutes to spare, nothing makes me feel better than going through a drawer and reorganizing it. Think of all the cabinets, closets, and purses that will benefit.

SHOP OR SELL ONLINE Need a gift for someone who's hard to buy for? You'll probably find the perfect item on the Web; clean out your attic and get some cash for your trash.

Most people who struggle with weight loss have turned eating into a hobby, something to do to keep busy and occupied. Breaking a habit and substituting another for it typically takes about thirty days, though for one as ingrained as eating all the time, it can easily take longer for the impulse to stop "pestering" you. But *it can be done.*

oh rats!

B. F. Skinner (1904–1990) was a highly influential though controversial American psychologist. His experiments with behavioral reinforcement in rats can teach us a lot as we seek to break unwanted eating habits.

Skinner's rats were all taught that pressing a bar in their cage released a food pellet. They associated pressing the bar with satisfying their physical hunger. Then, for some rats, Skinner made the bar work only intermittently. The rats learned that if they kept pressing, eventually they would be rewarded with food. For the intermittent rats, even when the bar stopped working completely, because of the off-again, on-again conditioning, they kept pressing the bar for a long time. Somewhere inside they knew if they kept it up, they'd get the food eventually, even after hundreds of presses, days of presses, with no reward. The rats whose bars worked one day and then the next day stopped working permanently learned very quickly not to press the bar. Once the reward was taken away, the association between the action and food was broken in a relatively short time.

I don't know about you, but if I want to break a habit (such as not eating in front of the evening news or not buying malted milk balls when I walk past the vendor at the mall), I'm much more successful if I stop completely. It hurts for a little while, and then it is truly broken. If I give in every other time that I have the desire, it only makes the battle longer and more painful.

Make your own list of activities to try the next time you want to chow down. And then try the *STOP* technique:

See whether the hunger is "head" or "physical."
Talk through your current situation or emotions before eating.
Organize a list of other possible activities.
Practice something else on your list.

Activities List

_____

_____

_____

_____

_____

_____

_____

_____

_____

_____

not "no" but "later"

Sometimes the best way to handle temptation is simply to delay—to say not "No" but "Later."

Let's face it, there will be days when sticking with our diets is harder than others because life is stressful or you're just plain ravenous for some reason. Forget the behavior modification and eating on the lower end of your calories. Some days we just need to make it through with all our "free food," extra points, and load-up items. But then there are the days when we feel more in control. Those are great times to work on changing old habits.

Here's an example: You're going along minding your own ̸
when all of a sudden you want a bag of 94 percent fat-free pop̸
you just had lunch. You stop and evaluate and know you're not ̸
hungry. But you have plenty of calories left and you really wa̸
are you going to do? Challenge yourself. Try walking away ̸̸
while. Say, "I'm going to go finish that closet or write my report or weed the garden. When I'm done, if I still want it, I'm going to eat some pop-corn."

You'll be amazed how many times you will get busy and forget the popcorn—and not think about it again until much later. Learning that you *can* walk away is exciting, empowering, and vitally important to long-term success. Give it a try!

keep yourself motivated all the way

Not long ago, years after I lost all my weight, a woman from my neighborhood stopped by. We were always friendly but had never been close. Our children were different ages and we just chatted from time to time when we caught each other in the street or the yard.

She was so sweet. She came over to apologize, saying that she had purposely snubbed me for the last few years. She had seen me in the yard and, not knowing who I was, thought Mark had dumped "me" and had gotten a new wife. Then, after reading an article about me, she realized what had happened—I was the other woman!

I couldn't believe it! I laughed, gave her a hug, and told her how much I appreciated her standing up for what she thought was a terrible thing that had happened to me.

Thanks, Marianne! You gave me one more little nugget that I can use in the future when, in a moment of insanity, I may start to wonder if what I've accomplished really feels better than eating. This does!

Sticking to your program for weeks, months, and years may seem at first to be mostly about the food you eat, but you and I both know that sustaining weight loss requires as much mental effort as it does physical. When I speak about losing weight and keeping it off, one of my most-asked questions is, "How did you stay motivated for *two years?*"

Here's how I respond: "Two years? I've had to stay motivated a lot longer than two years!" Sure, I needed to stay motivated to lose the weight, but if I didn't keep myself motivated *after* reaching goal, I knew I would put it all back on . . . and then some. You'll always need to find some way of motivating yourself—and you have to learn how to renew and refresh that motivation all the time.

Motivation is personal. Sometimes you're motivated to lose weight because of an upcoming event—a wedding, a class reunion, something like that. But what do you do the day after? Let yourself go back to where you were?

As you read this chapter, think about what motivates you. This will provide you with powerful information, which is the key to succeeding over time to lose the weight and keep it off.

Do you respond to positive motivation? Does your refrigerator feature a beautiful photo of you when you were wearing your favorite little black dress? Or do you need reminders of where you don't want to be by posting the nasty photo that sent you rushing to join a weight loss support group?

For most people, it's a combination of both. A dose of negative reality, such as hearing from your doctor that your cholesterol is very high, can certainly frighten you into immediate action. But focusing on the negative can be debilitating, even depressing—and although it may have gotten you to the starting gate, it's unlikely to fuel you through your weight loss journey. Instead, you may start thinking, "Why bother? I know I'll *never* be able to change anyway."

You need to banish those negative voices so that positive, encouraging messages fill your head.

Alan just finished writing his third-grade speech on Thomas Edison and the lightbulb. My favorite part of his speech was when he quoted Edison, saying, "I have not failed. I have found ten thousand ways that did not work!"

making motivation last

When we first start a new diet plan, we're excited, determined to make it work. It's like that feeling of being in a new relationship. It's all fresh and even kind of fun. You're feeling good about what you're doing. You're losing weight and feeling strong. I call this the honeymoon phase, when

> ## The only way you'll *never* lose weight
> ## is if you stop trying.

you're in love with your diet and nothing can distract you from your commitment. Wouldn't it be great if we could keep the honeymoon going all the way to goal? Steady weight loss, positive attitude—could anything be better? Wouldn't it be wonderful if you could make it last?

Then it happens. You get an undeserved zapping from the scale god. Or you've got a party nearly every night during the holidays. Or your kids are sick. It's been raining for days. The store doesn't have your favorite cereal, the one you depend on! You're tired of salad. You miss lasagna. Your pals are going out to the Cheesecake Factory. The weekend is coming. You're going on vacation. You lost your job. Your cat dies. Your dad dies.

Pick one. Any one.

These are all reasons why emotional eaters turn to food. *Do we really need a good reason?* Any of them are possible, and some may happen to you simultaneously. If nothing on the list happens to you, something similar or worse probably will.

How do I know? Because that is life. We all have to cope with stressful problems, invitations, family issues—*life.* Sometimes it's better. Sometimes it's worse. But life—the surprises, the challenges, the sorrows, the joys—happens.

The goal is learning how to "do life" without using food to manage it.

Every time you have a fight with your boyfriend, do you devour a pint of Ben & Jerry's Chocolate Chocolate Chunk? And does it help? I already know the answer to that one . . .

Well, chances are good you haven't had your last spat. But swallowing more than a thousand calories to make yourself feel better won't do the trick. In fact, it will only make you feel worse.

change it up

When I weighed more than three hundred pounds, I didn't leave the house more than I had to. It was my safe place, where no one could see or criticize me. It was easier to stay home instead of exhausting myself by moving through the ordinary activities of daily life. I did what I had to do, but I didn't do much more.

Once I began losing weight, I needed to find ways to break my bad habits and start new ones. By paying close attention to the triggers I felt, I realized that there were two times of day when I really thought about food a lot—the afternoon and the evening. (I know, I know, that is most of the day, but that is how it was for me in the beginning.)

My life consisted of so many food-centered routines and habits that I really needed a physical change to deal with some of them. I needed to get out of the house with my two little guys for the afternoon. I would pack them up and head to the movies (I brought my own popcorn), a museum, or the mall (I carried planned and measured snacks to have there).

I window-shopped and watched the kids in the playland while I wrote in my journal or planned another day's meals. Sometimes I'd leave the house to do errands that would take half the afternoon or head to my friend Cathy's house, where the kids could play while we encouraged and motivated each other.

If you're stuck at home during the day with kids, you know what I was up against—and why I had to get out of the house. The change in environment meant a chance to put old habits aside and structure a new routine that worked for my weight loss.

Evenings were hard, too. In the beginning, I found it so tough, I decided to go to bed with the boys around 8 p.m. I would take a favorite book and a cup of hot tea and brush my teeth and fall asleep reading. I got more sleep in those first months than I ever had, and I felt just wonderful.

Heading for bed early meant there were fewer hours to deal with those old food messages. Instead of struggling to resist them, I shut them down by shutting my eyes—and it worked for me. Yes, I got a little less done than I was used to doing, but when I calculated the impact on my improved health and break of poor habits, the time was well spent. I didn't do it forever, either—just for a time. And the payback was huge!

When I started staying up later with Aleeta, Adam, and Mark, I kept my hands busy crocheting while they did homework and watched the news. If they wanted a snack, I asked them to keep the food in the kitchen, which they were happy to do. From then on, I rarely ate after dinner—even now, I don't plan an evening snack very often. It's not like I still fight it every night. Those habits truly are broken. I hardly ever think about eating in the evening any more.

all or nothing

I enjoy crocheting. I always complete my projects and they look lovely. If I drop a stitch, even many rows back, I can rip out the stitches, stick my needle in the loop, and continue on.

But I don't seem to be able to knit. Oh, I can go through the motions, knit one, purl two, and complete a row. In fact, I've knitted entire rows that appear neat and even. But by the time I get to the sixth or seventh row, I notice that the width of my scarf is narrower than when I first started. I can't figure out where those stitches went and how to get them back.

Unless I can knit perfectly from beginning to end, without making one mistake or missing one stitch, I will never finish my scarf. It's so discouraging. I get a quarter of the way there and have to rip out my scarf back to the beginning and start all over again. This struggle has kept me from ever being able to complete one knitting project.

It's a lot like weight loss. You start out perfectly, feeling "This is it! I'm going to do it this time." You purge your cupboards of all those tempting food items and stock your refrigerator with healthy, low-fat treats. You plan your first day, make a bowl of sugar-free Jell-O, and pack a healthy lunch.

You buy some new workout clothes (because the elastic has disintegrated from the waistband of the last pair of sweats). You stock your gym bag with new pocket-sized shampoos and deodorants and invest in that pricey, really cool water bottle. *Ta da!* You've cast your stitches and you're on your way. *Knit one.*

Day after day, you stick with it. This isn't as hard as you thought! Why didn't you do it sooner?! People begin noticing you're losing weight. Woo-hoo! This is actually fun. *Purl two.*

And then—work is unusually busy and you forgot to pack your lunch. You stop at the store for necessities and grab some low-calorie cookies to nibble on. Somehow, as you're shopping, the entire bag disappears! How did *that* happen? You look under the cart. No cookies there. There's no way you finished all those cookies, did you? What have you *done*? You're angry. Disappointed. Still hungry. Unprepared and tired, you continue your pity binge. As long as you're "off" your diet, you may as well have a pizza and those Yodels you've been craving as well.

Back home, in bed for the night, you feel the tears running down your cheeks. *Why?* After all those weeks of work, why? You vow you'll get back on track tomorrow.

But tomorrow comes and your confidence is shaken. It's not as easy to hop back on as you thought. Today is weigh-in and you don't want your record book to show a gain. You decide to wait until next week. Instead of going to the support meeting you need the most, you skip it and flounder some more.

Remember my knitting analogy? You've dropped a stitch in your scarf and can't seem to pick it up again. You continue to unravel stitch after stitch. Your weight climbs and before long, you've unraveled back to the beginning. You'll have to make the scarf another day. You roll up the ball of yarn, stick in the needles, shove it in the back of the closet, and shut the door.

It doesn't have to be that way!

Knitting is *not* an impossible skill to learn—even after years of trying. Neither is weight loss. I cast my stitches one more time in 2001. With two hundred pounds to lose, I never thought I'd finish, but two years after I began, I was done.

I dropped some stitches along the way, but I learned how to unravel only to the dropped stitch, not all the way to the beginning. *You can, too.*

It's taken me a while, but since that fateful cookie episode, I've learned to retrain my "all-or-nothing" personality. Yes, I still slip up every now and then. *Everybody does.* We're human. The difference is, now I have the tools to be able to put the brakes on—and not let a slip turn into a slide all the way down to the bottom.

Instead of feeling helpless and falling, dig in your heels and get back to the basics. You know what works, so do it—and you'll make a fresh start.

five steps to recovering from a slip-up

1. *Stop!* Clean the house! What I mean is, go through your home, your office, and your car—and throw out anything that isn't part of your plan. Throw it away. Stop the madness. Don't worry about wasting food. Remember, it's either *waste* or *waist*! Which do you want?

2. *Plan! Plan! Plan!* Take the time to write out your food plans for the next few days. Or find your old ones. (You were saving them, right?) Look them over. This is *key*!

3. *Prepare.* Make a trip to the store and stock your the house with anything you're going to need. Buy lots of prepared vegetables if you're too busy to cut them up. Pick up a new journal or tracking system to reflect your fresh start. *Get ready!*

4. *Ask for help.* Tell the people who support you that you feel a little out of control. Think of things they can do to help. Maybe they've been part of the problem—inviting you out for too many restaurant meals. Figure out what you need and ask for it, or you're unlikely to get it!

5. *Do it!* Remember that wonderful Nike campaign? *Just do it.* It takes two to three tough days of sticking to your food plan to get that WOW! feeling back. But it does come back. (Really! Trust me.) You will experience that honeymoon feeling again, and it won't take long. But don't do it partway. Don't do it sloppy. Take it meal by meal. Snack by snack. Remember—you only have to do it for today . . . *every day.*

You have to learn to do this Five-Step Recovery Process, because you will *always* have to do it. Perfection isn't possible, but long-term weight loss and maintenance are. Every person who loses a lot of weight and maintains it has to regroup from time to time and find fresh motivation.

Practice these steps, and anytime you slip, you can use them to get back in the groove. That's what successful dieting is all about. (Hint: That's what maintenance is all about, too.)

Which brings me to the next source of motivation—or heartbreak: *the scale.*

all hail the scale

I lead a weight loss meeting one night each week. As much as my members and I love each other, I know it's not me they come to see—it's . . . the scale!

You'd be amazed at how many items people take off when they get weighed (or maybe you wouldn't). There are the normal things like belts, watches, and wallets. But some people divest themselves of much smaller items like bobby pins, toe rings, earrings—even tiny ones. One member won't even put on her paper nametag until after being weighed!

I've seen people drop their sweaters—and their pants! And I don't even bother to offer low-fat food samples to anyone waiting in line anymore. Eat something right before weigh-in? *Are you kidding?*

While they're waiting in line to get weighed, I greet the members and ask how they are. Inevitably, I get answers like, "I'll let you know in a minute." "Ask me again after I'm weighed." Or "I'm not sure, I haven't been weighed in yet."

> Never give up. Never give up. Never give up.
> —*Winston Churchill*

If I sound amazed, I'm not. I've been in that line myself many times. I know exactly what they mean. My own weight losses and gains still have an effect on my emotions. If I'm up a few pounds for no apparent reason, I feel frustrated and discouraged. If my weight stays the same after a week's vacation, I'm elated. Up. Down. Fear. Joy. It's amazing the power we allow the scale to wield over our lives.

I often have to remind myself that the scale is going to have only as much power as I give it. What is the scale, after all? It is a measuring device of our body's weight during that brief nanosecond in time. *It can't even differentiate between fat and water weight!* You may have actually lost fat during the week and yet still see an increase on the scale. It's influenced by any number of things: when you went to the bathroom last, what you ate or drank right before weigh-in, or how much sodium you recently consumed. That's not to mention the hormonal shifts that affect so many women throughout their lives.

As the leader of this group, I observe a range of emotions at the weigh-in—frustration, fear, victory, disappointment, excitement. It's all there. But let's face it—we give the scale more power over our emotional well-being than it deserves!

You could try to ignore it. But everywhere you go, those numbers on the scale provide an uncomfortable reminder. You fill out an insurance form and have to check off a weight range. You go for a doctor's visit and the first thing you have to do is to step on the scale. Even purchasing a pair of pantyhose requires knowing your weight (a good reason for never asking a guy to pick up a pair for us!)

We measure the progress of our diets by the numbers on the scale. For that brief moment in time, this is what *this* machine on *this* particular floor in a room with *this* specific air pressure says. *That's it.* Nothing more.

The scale can't measure behavior or determination, two things that are much more important to long-term weight loss than the numbers themselves. So the scale *cannot* be the only measure we use to feel successful.

There *will* be weeks when you do everything perfectly—plan and pre-

If I got on the scale and weighed 136 pounds, then stepped off the scale and drank a pint of water (remember, a pint is a pound) and stepped back on the scale, what would the scale say? 137, right! Does that mean I would be a pound heavier? Think now. The answer is yes. I would be a pound heavier. But that pound would be very temporary. It was a pound of water weight and would be gone in about an hour (or less). Think about it. The scale really is a very inaccurate measure of how we've done. Remember that.

pare and weigh and measure and exercise and stick like glue—and the scale stays the same, or (horror of horrors) goes up! *Eeeeeeeek!*

It's hard to accept that our bodies aren't machines that always behave exactly the same way, even if we do exactly the same thing to them. There are a myriad of reasons—cycles and hormones and medication and bloating among them—that the scale doesn't show a weight loss. And though the slight gain may be temporary, its power to shatter your motivation and confidence can be devastating.

finding motivation away from the scale

What can you do when the scale lets you down?

Well, let's think about what really motivates you. Sure, it's great to be able to see lower numbers on the scale, but the numbers aren't really the reason we want to lose weight, right? Who knows the numbers anyway, besides our doctors and ourselves? No. It's not *the numbers*. It's what comes along with them. Take some time to make a list of all the reasons you want to lose weight. There should be a lot of them, and it can be very motivational! Here are a few ideas:

your health

Blood pressure—Losing weight will help you lower it to normal.

Heart—It won't have to work so hard!

Cancer—Eating a healthy diet may protect you from some forms of cancer.

Blood sugar—Wouldn't it be great to have a low number?

Osteoporosis—Healthy eating keeps bones strong.

More energy—You won't be carrying as much weight around.

Less winded—Breathe free!

Aches and pains—You're likely to hurt a lot less when your muscles don't have so much weight to support.

Get off some medications—Losing weight may decrease your need for some medicines.

Feel better—Your body will thank you!

Live longer!—And feel better the longer you live!

your family

Be around for your spouse and children.

Set a good example for others you love.

Be more active and have more fun.

Be able to participate in their lives more.

your job

You have less need for extra sick days.

You can be more competitive for new jobs.

You'll be more confident with potential clients.

yourself

One size in your closet . . . a smaller one!

Everything fits . . . in styles you like.

You can cross your legs.

Painting your toenails and putting on panty hose or socks or shoes is easier.

You can buckle up in a car or on an airplane.

You can wear over-the-counter jewelry.

You can fit into your old jeans.

You'll feel the satisfaction of accomplishment.

You'll have increased self-confidence and pride.

Make a list of the things that *you* want that mean the most to *you:*

_____

_____

_____

_____

_____

_____

_____

_____

Keep this list close to you. Make multiple copies of it. Store it on your computer in case you misplace it. It may be your most valuable tool on your weight loss journey—especially when you have a rough week or make some bad choices. Looking at this list will be a good reminder of *all* the reasons you want to stick with your program, not just for the numbers on the scale.

When the scale does let you down, take a minute to reflect on all the nonscale victories you've had as well. Better health can't always be measured in pounds, but it can be measured. And seeing the progress can be *very* motivational.

Give yourself a nonscale check-up. Here are six other ways to motivate yourself when the scale disappoints you:

✓ *Check out your closet.* Have you been able to go "shopping" there since starting your new food regimen? See how close you are to zipping up those beloved jeans you haven't worn in years.

✓ *Check out the numbers.* Not the ones on the scale, but the other important numbers. Have you had your cholesterol checked lately? Measured your blood sugars or blood pressure? Compare your current measurements to the ones you wrote in your journal when you began. (Another great reason to journal.)

✓ *Check out your energy.* Are you huffing and puffing less going up and down the stairs? Are you able to walk further and faster? Can you keep up with your kids or grandkids or co-workers better?

✓ *Check out your emotions.* You've been working hard at making many lifestyle changes. Have you noticed a boost in your self-esteem and confidence levels along with a better body image? Feeling more positive about life in general?

✓ *Check out physical changes.* Have your sleep patterns improved? Are your aches and pains diminishing? Have your heartburn and indigestion lessened? What can your body do now that it couldn't before? *I loved it when I could finally cross my legs!*

✓ *Have YOU been checked out lately?* Has anyone been complimenting you about how good you look? When I had more than two hundred pounds to lose, people weren't sure about my weight loss at first, but they knew *something* looked better. Those comments are so rewarding!

Remember what the scale can't do:

The scale *can't* measure your will, your drive, how much time you put into your food plan, or how many temptations you said no to. It *can't* tell how many old habits you broke or new, healthier habits you started. It *doesn't* know the effort you put in at the gym, and it doesn't care. It *won't* heap praise on you because you chose the stairs over the elevator, or know that you passed on a slice of a colleague's birthday cake even though you wanted it with all your heart.

Most of all, the scale doesn't have any idea how hard you're trying, or how many times you overcame a slip and got back on track when you felt like giving up all together. *Only you know that.*

Every time you get on the scale, take a minute to measure what's *really* important, especially your behavior and your effort. We all get zapped by the scale from time to time. It's inevitable. But even if you feel as if the scale gave you a D for weight this week, give yourself an A for effort when you've had a fabulously successful week. I promise you, that effort *will* show up at the scale eventually.

The first time I was on the *Today* show, Natalie Morales asked me, "So what do you do when you've had a bad weigh-in?" I told her what I'll tell you now. After each weigh-in, you always have two choices: You can keep going or you can quit.

Remember, the only way you'll never lose weight is if you stop trying.

take the hit

When everything is going just fine, you can't wait to see what the scale says—you deserve to see a nice loss, right? But what if you overate on a couple of days this week? What if you succumbed to a piece of cake at a party, or an extra glass of wine? You think, *Oh no! What have I done? I can't go to my meeting and get on that scale. What if I don't lose this week or show a gain? I can't have that!*

So you decide to skip the meeting, wait till next week, and lose the weight you may have gained before going back. You want to have a perfect record book, right? You certainly wouldn't want those receptionists to give you that knowing look or that glance of concern and empathy.

So instead of going when you need the encouragement most, you fearfully forge ahead on your own. (It's like saying that you have to clean your house before the cleaning lady arrives or do your hair in order to go to the beauty parlor. It's crazy!)

Don't do it this time!

Not one of us will have a perfect record going from fat to finally thin. I know this may be hard for you, but please, if and when you have a difficult week, take the hit and keep on going. Don't they say that 80 percent of success is just showing up?

You can handle the truth. It's all part of life. No one is going to go from A to Z, from overweight to thin, in one straight line. Learn how to unravel, hop back on, and keep on going.

Take charge of your weight loss and don't let the scale dictate what you do and feel. Keep going. Keep showing up. Your future happiness really does depend on it!

patience: why it's a virtue

"Are we there yet?"

These words echo in my brain. The only downside to our treks to Maine are these four words. I cringe when they're first uttered by my seven-year-old or his nine-year-old brother—somewhere around Sturbridge, Massachusetts—only because I know it's the beginning of the end.

I know that they're really not asking if we're at our destination. It's pretty evident that we're not. We're still in the car, driving on a highway, not on a ferry on the way to Peaks Island, or even pulling into the harbor's parking garage.

They're just stating the simple fact that they're sick and tired of being on the same monotonous journey and they want their freedom. They want out, plain and simple.

My response is key. If I just say, *"No!"* and try to ignore them, it won't be long before they ask again. If, however, I say, "Not yet," and also ask if they'd like to play the alphabet game with me or spot unusual buildings along the way, we can actually make it clear to Portsmouth, New Hampshire, my two distracted little boys pressing their noses against the windows and never realizing we're still not "there" yet.

Isn't this a lot like a weight loss journey? We start out with great excitement and eagerness. But before long, monotony, boredom, and frustration with our lack of freedom set in.

Are we there yet?

We want out, plain and simple!

The feelings are legitimate—and the solution much the same. Rather than just saying *"No!"* and toughing it out to the end—or even worse, never making it at all—how much better it is to find simple distractions or notice exciting new sights that can make the journey more enjoyable.

What can you do to make your weight loss journey more exciting? Time is going to pass anyway, and because you're doing this for a lifetime, you need to work at keeping yourself interested and motivated. Here are a few ideas to help:

- Head to the library to check out a few light cookbooks.

- Check out the bookstore for a new planner or other weight loss tracking tool.

- Go to the grocery store to check out a new light product you've heard about and want to try.

- Get to your gym and schedule an hour with one of the trainers.

- Visit the fanciest store in town and see if you can slip into some of the fashions that are way out of your price range.

- Have your nails done (it's harder to eat Oreos that way).

- Have your teeth whitened.

The list can go on and on. See how many ideas you can generate!

Look for ways to break up the monotony and increase your pleasure in the journey. And the next time you ask, "Are we there yet?" the answer will be *Yes!*

There's no getting around it—dieting takes patience. When I had more than two hundred pounds to lose, I didn't spend much time looking ahead and figuring out when I might reach my goal. It just seemed way too far away. But as I got closer, I began to calculate when it might happen. As my weight loss slowed, I felt so impatient—and even a little worried. Maybe I wouldn't get there after all.

Weight loss is never a steady course. Some months you lose more than you expected; some months you lose less than you hoped. If you map out the monthly estimates of what you expect to lose and don't make it, you may see it as a failure—rather than *celebrating* the weight you did lose. Don't let it get you off track!

There is very little difference in what you need to do to lose one pound of fat, compared to 212 pounds of fat. *It's the same thing 212 times.* The difference is only the amount of time you need to stay motivated.

But if you're going to be doing it forever anyway, it doesn't matter whether you reach goal in September or December or the spring. Focus on daily living—finding supreme enjoyment in your new lifestyle, not how quickly you can hit the number and end the diet.

Whether you have a few pounds to lose or a few hundred, enjoy your daydreams about reaching goal—but recognize that they are just that, daydreams. When you're done say, "Okay, what can I do *today* to make that happen?"

The more effort you put into *today,* the more you plan and prepare for *today,* the more you focus on *today,* the more likely it is that you'll reach that goal tomorrow!

make it for life— maintenance

Journal entry: June 2005

"Living" on a diet has many rewarding moments, and many that are frustrating and painful. It's never-ending. Do you ever wonder if it'll be worth it?

Right now I'm in our road-worn minivan with two overtired boys and a carsick puppy at my feet. I have one eye on my husband, who still has four hours of driving as I type away on my laptop and hope my battery holds out. We've just spent three beautiful days visiting my parents on Peaks Island off the coast of Portland, Maine.

Island life is lovely in midspring. Year-round residents break forth from their homes to spruce up yards, clean up storefronts, and paint the underbellies of their boats before the summer guests arrive. This morning the waterfront ice cream parlor opened its doors for the season. Children lined up, hoping to be the first customer of the season. It was fun to be part of this time-honored tradition. I ordered a cone along with everyone else and was glad the owners had low-fat vanilla. It wasn't sugar-free, but I had planned a low-calorie meal for later in the day.

The kids scootered home ahead of us. While we reminisced about opening days gone by, I was mentally working out the new fat-free fettuccine recipe I planned to serve for lunch. These small cones wouldn't hold us for long.

For my part, the weekend hadn't been an easy one. Mom, who usually stocks her home with my favorite diet beverages and fat-free snacks, had been sick the week before and wasn't her usual prepared self. Every time I turned around to fix something that was "on my diet," a key ingredient was missing. Sometimes I skipped. Sometimes I substituted a higher-fat version and just had a smaller portion. It was frustrating to be working this hard, eating less than usual, and knowing I was still over my calorie limit. With each meal I had to readjust my plan. And with each recipe my efforts were thwarted. At one time in my life I would have just given up, thinking it just wasn't worth it.

The next day as we walked to the ferry to begin our trek home, I was reminded that I couldn't always make this trip on foot. At 350 pounds, I used to have to be driven while everyone else walked. I felt a moment of intense gratitude for my healthy body. It was a great reminder to savor each victory and deal with each frustration the best I could. In the end, I decided as I walked to the ferry without huffing and puffing, it was definitely worth it.

Now it's time for us to talk about the impossible dream for so many dieters—life on maintenance. If you've purchased this book, you've probably been disappointed in your efforts to maintain your weight loss goal in the past. But this time is going to be different.

what is maintenance?

I looked it up in the dictionary. To maintain is "to keep something in existence or continuance." Okay, but let's keep going. I want to know more.

Webster defines *continuance* as "To go on after interruption. To keep on, to last or endure, to remain in a place; abide; stay."

That's it!

Maintenance is staying with it, enduring through thick and thin, keeping on keeping on.

Maintenance is for **LIFE.**

Long-term
Investment
Focused
Enjoyment

> You don't have to do this *forever.*
> You just have to do this *for today.* Every day.

long-term

"How long do you think this will *take*?" People ask me that all the time when they start a new weight-loss program. Here's my answer: "It *takes* everyone exactly the same amount of time . . . the rest of our lives."

When, along that path, do I think they'll hit goal? No one knows for sure. It depends on your metabolism, how far you have to go, and how hard you work at it. But asking how long it will *take* suggests that there is an end. And that's not the way we want to be thinking.

It doesn't matter whether you are starting a diet for the first, twentieth, or umpteenth time; whether you lose slowly now that you're older and less active; whether you need a guide to follow to make sure you're eating healthy; or whether you've lost the same forty-five pounds over and over again your whole life. We all will be "on" this for the rest of our lives—or we will continue to yo-yo and feel the pain.

Understanding that is what made the difference for me between all the partially used membership books in my nightstand and a 212-pound weight loss. I know what it's like to give up. I also know how to succeed. It's never over—but it does get easier. You just have to accept that you're in it for the *long term.*

investment

This is no small thing you have accomplished. Of the sixty-five million Americans who are on a diet at any given day, you are in the small percentage who made it to goal. Now let's stay there—and keep you in the small percentage (2 to 5 percent) who *don't* gain the weight back! That will take ongoing work and continued investment in your future.

But you've already proved that you can do it. Here are some tips to help *keep* you doing it. It's kind of like your investment portfolio—designed to pay off in big dividends:

- *Weigh yourself* at least once each week. This is one way of knowing whether your weight is creeping back up. *Don't let the scale get ahead of you.* If you see that the numbers are going in the wrong direction and you know your eating is getting off track, head back to step 9—and reclaim your motivation with the Five-Step Recovery Process.

• *Once you reach goal, increase your daily calories* by about 50 for the first week. (Consult your diet plan if its maintenance advice differs.) Weigh yourself again. If you continue to lose weight, increase your daily calories again by 50–75 for the next week. And so on until you stop losing. If you see a gain, you can decrease your daily calories a little. At some point your body will find a comfortable set point. That will be your target calorie range.

• *Keep a daily journal* of your food plans and anything else you find helpful. It will be a terrific resource as you track and evaluate your maintenance experience.

• *Continue using your support systems.* Whether you've chosen support that's online, in person, professional, or through family and friends, it will be at least as important now as when you were losing your weight. After all those compliments about your hard work, after being held up as an example to others, you may find it hard to show your vulnerability, but as anyone who has ever lost weight and gained it back knows, maintenance is a very precarious time. Use your support and *ask* for help when needed!

• *As you weigh in each week, it's also a good time to weigh your feelings and actions.* Take two minutes to evaluate your actions. Are some of your old "bad" habits creeping back in? Are you succumbing to those BLTs (Bites, Licks, and Tastes)? Are you getting sloppy in your eating habits? Not planning? Overindulging more often? How do you feel physically? Still full of vim and vigor? Or are you getting a little sluggish and lacking your newfound energy? Watch the scale, but listen to your body as well.

• *Keep it up or ramp it up.* If you haven't been consistent in your exercise, there's no time like maintenance to kick up that part of your new lifestyle. It will give you something new and exciting to focus on. Make that a strong part of your *SIMPLE* goals for the future. If you *have* incorporated exercise into your new lifestyle, *great*! Think about how you can ramp it up. Maybe it's time to make an appointment with a personal trainer as a reward for your new weight loss. Wherever you're at in your activity and exercise program, it can be a great time to push for new challenges. Adding to your workout, perhaps by increasing your strength workout sessions, can work wonders on your metabolism during your maintenance.

- *Plan and prepare* now more than ever. Make sure those cupboards stay stocked with foods that keep you on track. Don't let red-light foods creep in. Keep searching out new light products at the supermarket, and keep lightening up those family favorites. Remember, 200 little calories each day more than your body needs adds up to twenty pounds gained each year!

focused

The excitement is gone. No more losses at the scale to look forward to. No more anticipation of new sizes. No more comments about how great you look or "How did you ever do it?!" All that's left is . . . living this "diet" for the rest of your life . . . *without* the fun perks! How are you going to do it?

Part of maintenance is simply making sure your weight is still on your radar. The goal is for your diet to become your way of life. Making it second nature to you is a good thing. Being on autopilot simply means you're walking the walk. But as your comfort level increases, so does the danger that old habits will creep back in.

When you get to goal it is very easy to let the excitement of being at this lovely new size blind you to the fact of how easy it is for it to slip away. I have a very healthy respect for where I could go again if I let my guard down. Do you? Haven't you gained the weight back enough times in the past? It might take a month to lose four to five pounds, but it's not hard to put it back on in a week or two. Unfair, I know. But it is what it is.

One of the best ways to offset that is to revisit your maintenance goals. Remember the *SIMPLE* goals from step 2? Make your goals *specific, in writing, measurable, possible, limited in time,* and *enticing.* What are they now, and how do they differ from weight loss goals?

These should be just an extension of your existing goals. You will want to have short-term goals and long-term goals, too. Once you get to maintenance, let this list be one of the first things you do . . . after your victory dance!

my simple goals for maintenance

_____

_____

_____

_____

_____

_____

_____

enjoyment

I won't lie to you. When I weighed 350 pounds, there was a lot about the way I was eating that I enjoyed. Of course I didn't like the way the weight made me look or feel, but I *did* enjoy eating a lot of good-tasting food . . . *frequently.*

The flip side is also true. I hated dieting not because I hated losing weight, but because I didn't like how little or what I was eating. If something was made low-fat or light—forget it! I wasn't about to put it in my mouth. Small portions only left me unsatisfied.

Enjoyment is the key. If you don't enjoy it, you won't keep doing it.

So what else do I enjoy now? I love the fact that for five years in a row I have only one size in my closet.

I love being photographed with my family—and no longer hiding behind anyone or anything.

If I find myself feeling hungry for something that I don't eat anymore, I start making a list of the things I enjoy now that I'm at goal—and the list goes on and on. I can't wait until you get to make your own list and

> Motivation is what gets you started.
> Habit is what keeps you going.
> —*Jim Ryun*

experience the supreme enjoyment of living in the moment, really being where you want to be.

If you are extremely overweight, remember, there is a real blessing to having a lot of weight to lose. Why? By the time you reach your goal, many of your new healthier habits will be ingrained because you've practiced them for a longer period of time. You'll be one step ahead in your maintenance.

snacks-a-million

Snacking wasn't smiled on while I was growing up. Oh, it wasn't totally forbidden, but it all depended on when we asked. If it was within two hours of a meal, my mom's favorite mantra was, "You'll ruin your appetite!"

Actually, healthy snacking can be wonderful for taking the edge off hunger, keeping your blood sugar level and your metabolism on the go. A well-timed snack can even help you make better food choices and practice portion control at meals. Most of us don't have to worry about spoiling our appetites, do we?

If you're in the habit of grabbing Fritos or Twizzlers and can't think of a healthy snack other than celery sticks, here are a few of my favorites:

~ 25-calorie snacks

- a whole pack of sugar-free Jell-O (cut the water in half to make Jigglers)
- 4 ounces tomato or V8 juice with a celery stick garnish
- 1 cup air-popped popcorn
- 1 clementine, 1 apricot, or 3 halves dried apricots
- 1 medium tomato, sliced and sprinkled with Splenda
- 4 large shrimp or 1 ounce turkey breast
- 3 tablespoons fat-free Cool Whip (yup, out of the tub!)

~ 50-calorie snacks

- 1 cup grapes (freeze them for an added treat)
- 5 mini-meringues

- 8 ounces cappuccino with fat-free milk

- 1 tablespoon sunflower seeds

- 1 small egg

- 1.5 ounces lobster or smoked salmon

- ½ cup yogurt, fat free and artificially sweetened

- 1 cup strawberries or ½ grapefruit

- 1 fat-free Fudgsicle

~ 100-calorie snacks

- NEW! Kim's Light Bagels, six varieties (www.kimslightbagels.com)

- ½ cup sugar-free pudding, made with skim milk

- Campbell's Soup, many varieties

- 6 saltine crackers with 2 teaspoons peanut butter

- ½ turkey sandwich with light bread, mustard, and veggies

- ⅙ sugar-free angel food cake (brands vary)

- ½ cup light ice cream (brands vary)

- ½ cup fat-free cottage cheese with pineapple

- 1 VitaMuffin or a VitaBrownie (yum!)

- 1 Biscotti Brothers chocolate almond biscotti

- ½ bag Jelly Belly sugar-free jelly beans

- Tyson Fajita Chicken Breast Strips (3 ounces)

- any 100-calorie snack pack

low-carb snacks

- a handful of almonds or sunflower seeds

- turkey and cheese roll-ups

- hard-boiled egg or deviled egg

- egg-and-cheese omelet

- string cheese

- Geraldine's Bodacious Cheese Straws

- mushrooms stuffed with sausage, garlic, red peppers, and cream cheese, heated

- celery with tuna or peanut butter

- a whole pack of sugar-free Jell-O (cut the water in half to make Jigglers)

- smoked salmon and cream cheese on cucumber slices

- lettuce roll-ups with luncheon meat, egg salad, or tuna salad

- BLT stackers with romaine lettuce as the bread

recipes

beverages

coffee freeze

A cool and refreshing way to get in one of your dairy . . . and less than 100 calories!

1 cup nonfat milk
3 cups ice chips
1¼ cups frozen fat-free whipped topping
1 small box fat-free, sugar-free vanilla pudding
1 tablespoon instant coffee

Put all ingredients in a blender and blend until smooth. Serve immediately.

Makes 4 servings; Serving size: 1 cup

PER SERVING: ■■

Calories: 93	Total Carbs: 19 g
Total Fat: 0 g	Dietary Fiber: 1 g
Cholesterol: 1 mg	Protein: 3 g
Sodium: 363 mg	Sugar: 3 g

caffé hollywood

4 cups nonfat milk
6 tablespoons unsweetened cocoa powder
6 tablespoons powdered sugar
1 teaspoon vanilla extract
10 tablespoons Kahlúa (coffee liqueur)
4 cups double-strength coffee (perk or instant)

Mix the milk, cocoa powder, powdered sugar, and vanilla in a saucepan and bring just to a boil, but don't allow it to boil. Add the Kahlúa and coffee. Make sure the coffee flavor comes through. Add additional cocoa powder and/or coffee, if necessary. Serve in a pedestal coffee mug. For a cool and refreshing treat, this can be served over ice cubes.

Makes 8 servings; Serving size: 1 cup

PER SERVING: ■■

Calories: 135	Total Carbs: 23 g
Total Fat: 1 g	Dietary Fiber: 1 g
Cholesterol: 2 mg	Protein: 5 g
Sodium: 69 mg	Sugar: 15 g

Top with fat-free whipped cream and a pinch of cocoa powder (not included in nutritional info).

faux orange julius

Does an Orange Julius bring back great mall memories? That may be an oxymoron if you're not much of a shopper, but if you are, you may have slurped down a few OJs in your day. Yes, it has orange juice as a base, but that doesn't mean it's a "healthy" choice. Now you can make yours at home for the same great flavor with added fiber and none of the fat!

8 ounces Tropicana® Trop50
1 teaspoon Benefiber®
1 medium banana
1½ cups ice chips
3 packets Splenda®
3 tablespoons fat-free half & half

Mix the Benefiber together with the orange juice first. Put all ingredients together in a blender and blend until smooth.

Makes 2 servings; Serving size: 16 ounces

PER SERVING: ■

Calories: 105	Total Carbs: 25 g
Total Fat: 0 g	Dietary Fiber: 4 g
Cholesterol: 1 mg	Protein: 2 g
Sodium: 38 mg	Sugar: 6 g

frozen virgin margarita

For our light margarita with a kick, add a shot of tequila. For each jigger (1.5 ounces) add 97 calories.

4 teaspoons Low-Calorie Granulated Sugar*
½ lime, cut into 4 wedges
2 tablespoons lime juice
½ cup light orange juice
1 package Crystal Light® Lemonade Mix
3½ cups crushed ice

Place the *Low-Calorie Granulated Sugar in a shallow dish. Rub the rim of each of 4 margarita glasses with a lime wedge and dip the rims into the sugar. Set the lime wedges aside.

In a blender, blend the lime juice, orange juice, lemonade mix, water, and ice on high speed for 1 to 2 minutes, or until well-blended. Enjoy!

Makes 4 servings; Serving size: 8 ounces

PER SERVING: ☐

Calories: 26	Total Carbs: 7 g
Total Fat: 0 g	Dietary Fiber: 0 g
Cholesterol: 0 mg	Protein: 0 g
Sodium: 6 mg	Sugar: 6 g

hot cocoa mix

Not many sugar-free hot chocolate mixes are rich *and* light.
Now you can make your own. This mix is great to make
ahead in bulk and store in an airtight container. Makes a
nice holiday gift, too.

2 tablespoons unsweetened cocoa powder
2 tablespoons sugar substitute
4 packs Splenda coffee flavoring, mocha
6 tablespoons instant nonfat dry milk

Mix all of the ingredients together. Place 2 tablespoons of the
mixture into a mug and fill with 10 ounces of boiling water.
Enjoy!

Makes 5 servings; Serving size: 2 tablespoons

PER SERVING: ☐

Calories: 23	Total Carbs: 5 g
Total Fat: 0 g	Dietary Fiber: 1 g
Cholesterol: 0 mg	Protein: 2 g
Sodium: 29 mg	Sugar: 3 g

Top with 1 candy cane or 25 mini-marshmallows for
an extra 70 calories.

kid's milkshake

My son, Alan, can't stand the texture of fruit but knows he has to eat it every day. We came up with this shake together, and it has made such a difference in the happiness level of the Bensen household every morning. Try it. You won't want to go out for fast-food, high-fat milkshakes any more!

1 large banana, 7-inch
1½ cups nonfat milk
3 tablespoons Hershey's sugar-free chocolate syrup
¼ teaspoon vanilla extract
1 cup crushed ice
2 packets sugar substitute
2 teaspoons Benefiber®

Put all of the ingredients in the jar of a blender. Cover and pulse for 90 seconds or until blended to desired consistency.

Makes 2 servings; Serving size: 12 ounces

PER SERVING ■■

Calories: 113	Total Carbs: 25 g
Total Fat: 0 g	Dietary Fiber: 3 g
Cholesterol: 0 mg	Protein: 8 g
Sodium: 98 mg	Sugar: 5 g

breads & brunch

banana bread

This is a slight variation on a recipe my mom got from her best friend, Marie Macomber, when they were young moms in Attleboro, Massachusetts. They've been baking this bread for years.

  Fat-free cooking spray
  1¾ cups all-purpose flour
  3 ripe medium bananas, mashed
  ¾ cup sugar substitute
  2¼ teaspoons baking soda
  4 ounces egg substitute
  ½ teaspoon salt

Preheat the oven to 325° F. Spray a loaf pan with fat-free cooking spray. Mix all of the ingredients using a food processor or an electric mixer. Pour the batter into the loaf pan. Bake for 1 hour, or until a toothpick inserted in the center comes out clean.

Makes 10 servings; Serving size: ¹/₁₀ of loaf

PER SERVING: ■■

Calories: 127	Total Carbs: 28 g
Total Fat: 1 g	Dietary Fiber: 1 g
Cholesterol: 2 mg	Protein: 4 g
Sodium: 252 mg	Sugar: 0 g

blueberry buckle

Our family members would do anything for one another. We give time, money, support in any way we can . . . Blueberry Buckle excluded. It's made at every family gathering but there's no grace when it comes to getting the last piece.

¾ cup low-calorie granulated sugar*
2 tablespoons Brummel & Brown® Spread
¼ cup Egg Beaters®
½ teaspoon vanilla
½ cup nonfat milk
2 cups cake flour
2 teaspoons baking powder
½ teaspoon salt
¾ cup unsweetened applesauce
2 cups fresh blueberries, washed

CRUMB TOPPING:

½ cup low-calorie granulated sugar*
⅓ cup cake flour
½ teaspoon cinnamon
¼ cup Brummel & Brown® Spread

Mix thoroughly the sugar, Brummel & Brown, Egg Beaters, and vanilla, and then stir in the milk. Mix together the flour, baking powder, and salt, and then stir in with the first mixture. Blend in applesauce and blueberries. Spray a 9-inch square baking dish with cooking spray and spread the batter in evenly.

Mix all the crumb topping ingredients together and sprinkle over the top of the blueberry mixture. Bake at 350°F for 45 to 50 minutes until toothpick thrust into center comes out clean.

Makes 16 servings; Serving size: ¹/₁₆ of recipe

PER SERVING: ■■

Calories: 111	Total Carbs: 32 g
Total Fat: 2 g	Dietary Fiber: 1 g
Cholesterol: 0 mg	Protein: 3 g
Sodium: 105 mg	Sugar: 18 g

blueberry muffins

I grew up raking blueberries on my great-grandfather's farm in Whiting, Maine—almost on the Canadian border. The blueberries there are tiny and as sweet as candy, and we always ate more than we took home.

Fat-free cooking spray
2½ cups all-purpose flour
2½ teaspoons baking powder
¾ cup sugar substitute
⅓ cup egg substitute
1 cup unsweetened applesauce
¾ cup nonfat milk
3¼ cups frozen unsweetened blueberries

Preheat the oven to 350° F. Spray a muffin tin with fat-free cooking spray or line with paper muffin liners. Mix the flour, baking powder, and sugar substitute in a large bowl. Mix the egg substitute, applesauce, and milk in a small bowl. Add to the dry ingredients and stir until blended. Fold in the blueberries. Spoon the batter into muffin cups. Bake for approximately 20 minutes.

Makes 12 servings; Serving size: 1 large muffin or 3 mini-muffins

PER SERVING: ■■

Calories: 134	Total Carbs: 30 g
Total Fat: 0 g	Dietary Fiber: 2 g
Cholesterol: 0 mg	Protein: 6 g
Sodium: 124 mg	Sugar: 6 g

breakfast burrito

A tasty, filling way to start the day!

½ cup egg substitute
¼ cup shredded fat-free Cheddar cheese
½ teaspoon sea salt
¼ cup salsa, chunky or smooth, hot or mild (you choose)
¼ cup diced green bell pepper
1 Kim's Light Flat Bread

Cook the egg substitute in a small nonstick frying pan. Once the egg starts to stiffen, add the cheese, salt, salsa, and bell pepper. Cook until the cheese is melted. Lay the filling evenly in the bread. Roll it up and cut it into 2 pieces. Enjoy!

Serve with a side of fruit for a beautiful and fiber-full breakfast.

Makes 2 servings; Serving size: ½ burrito

PER SERVING: ■■

Calories: 138	Total Carbs: 8 g
Total Fat: 3 g	Dietary Fiber: 2 g
Cholesterol: 3 mg	Protein: 15 g
Sodium: 1233 mg	Sugar: 1 g

broccoli and mushroom quiche

Great for breakfast or brunch, holidays or anytime.

CRUST:

Fat-free cooking spray
1¼ cups cooked brown rice, hot
¼ cup shredded low-fat Cheddar cheese

FILLING:

Two 10-ounce packages frozen chopped broccoli, thawed
1 cup canned sliced mushrooms, drained
6 ounces egg substitute
1 tablespoon salt
¼ cup shredded low-fat Cheddar cheese

Preheat the oven to 350° F. Spray a 9-inch pie pan with fat-free cooking spray. Mix together the hot brown rice and cheese and press into the pie pan. Mix the broccoli, mushrooms, egg substitute, and salt and pour into the crust. Bake for 45 minutes, or until well done. Turn off the oven. Sprinkle the quiche with the remaining cheese and return it to the oven for another 5 minutes to melt the cheese.

Makes 8 servings; Serving size: ⅛ of 9-inch quiche

PER SERVING:: ■■

Calories: 101	Total Carbs: 15 g
Total Fat: 1 g	Dietary Fiber: 3 g
Cholesterol: 3 mg	Protein: 8 g
Sodium: 477 mg	Sugar: 1 g

LOW-CARB OPTION: Eliminate the crust. It's not necessary for a delicious quiche and adds calories and carbs. Also try making this recipe in muffin tins for portioned mini-quiches that are great take-alongs. Total carbs: 3.7 grams.

corn bread

The sour cream makes it moist, but the corn makes it!

    Fat-free cooking spray
    2 packages Jiffy cornbread mix
    1 cup fat-free sour cream
    1/3 cup canned yellow sweet corn, drained
    3 ounces egg substitute
    1/4 cup fat-free milk

Preheat the oven to 400° F. Spray a 9 × 13-inch baking dish with fat-free cooking spray. Mix all of the ingredients in a medium bowl. Pour into the prepared dish and bake for 20 minutes, or until firm to the touch and light golden brown. Delish!

Makes 20 servings; Serving size: 1/20 of recipe

PER SERVING: ■■

Calories: 105	Total Carbs: 17 g
Total Fat: 2 g	Dietary Fiber: 0 g
Cholesterol: 2 mg	Protein: 2 g
Sodium: 230 mg	Sugar: 4 g

cobblestone

When I wrote *Finally Thin!* I would often sit at Panera for a little peace and quiet. Their rich baked goodies often tempted me, and, if I was ever looking to spend an extra 650 calories, I knew I could have chosen one of their Cobblestones. To be honest, that never happened, but it did inspire this delicious gooey breakfast treat . . . or dessert.

COBBLESTONE:

6 Kim's Light Bagels®* (plain, cinnamon, blueberry, or wheat)
1 cup Egg Beaters®
½ cup low-calorie powdered sugar* premixed with
   2 tablespoons water
1 teaspoon cinnamon

GLAZE:

¼ cup low-calorie powdered sugar*
2 teaspoons water

Chop the *Kim's Light Bagels into small pieces. Mix the Egg Beaters, ½ cup *Low-Calorie Powdered Sugar and water mixture, and the cinnamon. Blend well and evenly fill into the 6 sections of the Popover Pan. Bake at 350° F for 20 to 25 minutes until lightly browned.

For the glaze, mix the sugar and water. Drizzle over the cooled Cobblestones.

Makes 6 servings; Serving size: 1 cobblestone

PER SERVING: ■■

Calories: 155	Total Carbs: 48 g
Total Fat: 1 g	Dietary Fiber: 4 g
Cholesterol: 0 mg	Protein: 9 g
Sodium: 267 mg	Sugar: 24 g

eggcellent casserole

Amazingly light for such a hearty meal. Serve it anytime!

Fat-free cooking spray
Two 11-ounce packages low-fat Pillsbury Bread Sticks
½ cup shredded fat-free Cheddar cheese
2 cups egg substitute
1 teaspoon chipotle seasoning
2 teaspoons salt
1 teaspoon freshly ground black pepper
½ cup chopped red bell pepper
½ cup chopped green bell pepper
¼ cup chopped onion
½ cup sliced mushrooms

Spray a 9 × 13-inch baking dish with fat-free cooking spray. Roll 1 package of bread stick dough out flat to cover the bottom of the pan. Sprinkle with ¼ cup of the cheese. Roll out the other package of dough and lay it on top. Mix the egg substitute, chipotle seasoning, salt, and pepper, and pour on top of the dough. Add the bell peppers, onion, and mushrooms. Sprinkle the rest of the cheese on top. Cover and chill overnight.

Preheat the oven to 350° F. Bake for 45 to 50 minutes, or until a knife inserted in the center comes out clean.

Makes 16 servings; Serving size: ¹/₁₆ of recipe

PER SERVING: ■■

Calories: 97	Total Carbs: 14 g
Total Fat: 1 g	Dietary Fiber: 1 g
Cholesterol: 1 mg	Protein: 4 g
Sodium: 569 mg	Sugar: 2 g

garlic bagel bread

Finally . . . now you can have garlic bread without the guilt! This pull-apart garlic concoction is a fabulous compliment to all your Italian dishes.

¼ cup Brummel & Brown® Buttery Spread
5 garlic cloves, smashed and chopped
1 teaspoon sea salt
3 egg whites, scrambled
1 tablespoon Garlic Butter Seasoning*
2 teaspoons Tuscany Blend Italian Seasoning*
6 Kim's Light Bagels®*, chopped (use plain, onion, wheat, or everything)

In a skillet, cook Brummel & Brown, garlic cloves, and salt, and simmer 1 to 2 minutes over medium-high heat until Brummel & Brown is melted. In a bowl, combine scrambled egg whites, *Garlic Butter Seasoning and *Tuscany Blend Italian Seasoning. Toss egg-white mixture with *Kim's Light Bagels until combined. Pour butter-and-garlic mixture over bagels and toss lightly. Spread entire mixture into an ovensafe pie plate sprayed with fat-free cooking spray. Bake at 350°F for 20 to 25 minutes until golden brown.

Makes 8 servings; Serving size: ⅛ of recipe

PER SERVING: ■■

Calories: 120	Total Carbs: 18 g
Total Fat: 3 g	Dietary Fiber: 3 g
Cholesterol: 0 mg	Protein: 6 g
Sodium: 615 mg	Sugar: 1 g

monkey french toast

In the words of my little boys, "Yes!" This is ooey-gooey good.

Fat-free cooking spray
6 Kim's Light Cinnamon Bagels®*
1 cup egg substitute
1 teaspoon ground cinnamon
1 tablespoon sugar substitute
½ cup sugar-free maple syrup

Preheat the oven to 350°F. Spray a 9 × 13-inch baking dish with cooking spray. Cut the bagels into bite-size pieces. Mix all of the ingredients in a large bowl. Spread into the prepared pan and bake for 45 minutes.

Good topped with fat-free whipped cream or light ice cream, not factored. Garnish with a cinnamon-sugar substitute mix. You can slice and serve, or you can sit around the table and pull the pieces off and lick your fingers as you eat.

Makes 9 servings; Serving size: ⅑ of recipe

PER SERVING: ■

Calories: 90	Total Carbs: 16 g
Total Fat: 1 g	Dietary Fiber: 4 g
Cholesterol: 0 mg	Protein: 7 g
Sodium: 205 mg	Sugar: 1 g

popovers

The first time I had a popover was at David Burke's amazing
five-star restaurant in New York City. I fell in love that day.
Now you can make your own. Popovers are one of the most
versatile side breads (fill with chicken salad, ice cream, anything!) and are so easy to make. All you need is a popover
pan and a few basic ingredients.

1 egg
2 egg whites
1 cup nonfat milk
1 tablespoon Canola oil
1 cup all-purpose flour
½ teaspoon salt

Spray a Popover Pan* with nonstick spray. Beat egg and egg
whites until frothy; add in milk and oil and beat for another 3
minutes. Add flour and salt; beat until blended, about 30 seconds but still lumpy. Clean off sides of bowl and mix with a
spoon. Fill cups half full. Bake in 400°F oven until firm, allowing 25 minutes for pans or 30 minutes for muffin cups. Turn
off oven. Prick popovers with a fork. Leave in oven for 5 to 8
minutes more or until crispy. Serve warm.

Makes 6 servings; Serving size: 1 popover

PER SERVING: ■■

Calories: 122	Total Carbs: 18 g
Total Fat: 3 g	Dietary Fiber: 1 g
Cholesterol: 36 mg	Protein: 6 g
Sodium: 244 mg	Sugar: 0 g

appetizers & snacks

artichoke cups

An easy recipe that's a hit at the holidays . . . or any time of year. Love those wontons!

Fat-free cooking spray

24 wonton wrappers

¼ cup shredded fat-free Cheddar cheese

3 ounces fat-free cream cheese

½ teaspoon cayenne

2 teaspoons Dijon mustard

3 tablespoons diced red bell peppers

One 14-ounce can artichoke hearts in water, drained
and chopped

4 tablespoons chopped fresh parsley

Preheat the oven to 350° F. Prepare a miniature muffin pan by spraying it lightly with fat-free cooking spray. Gently press 1 wonton wrapper into each muffin cup, allowing the ends to extend above the cup. Lightly spray the edges of the wrappers with cooking spray and set aside. Combine the cheeses, cayenne, and mustard in a bowl and mix well. Stir in the bell peppers and artichoke hearts. Spoon about 1 heaping teaspoon of the cheese mixture into each muffin cup. Bake for about 15 minutes, or until the cheese mixture is set and the edges of the wrappers are lightly browned. Garnish with parsley and serve.

Makes 12 servings; Serving size: 2 tartlets

PER SERVING: ■

Calories: 64	Total Carbs: 11 g
Total Fat: 0 g	Dietary Fiber: 1 g
Cholesterol: 3 mg	Protein: 4 g
Sodium: 235 mg	Sugars: 0 g

artichoke dip

A high-fat version of this is served at the delightful Inn on Peaks Island off the coast of Portland, Maine. On Wednesday nights in the wintertime, they offer suppers for less than $8. Mark ordered hot artichoke dip once and I tasted it. I wanted to drown myself in it! This light version tastes just as delicious . . . but you don't get the ambiance!

One 14-ounce can artichoke hearts in water, drained
    and chopped
½ cup fat-free mayonnaise
1 medium sweet onion, minced
4 ounces light Jarlsburg cheese, cut into small pieces
8 ounces shredded fat-free mozzarella cheese

Preheat the oven to 375°F. Mix all of the ingredients in a small casserole or stoneware crock. Bake for 25 to 30 minutes, or until the cheese melts and bubbles. Serve with Kim's Light Bagel Chips (page 204).

Makes 12 servings; Serving size: ¼ cup

PER SERVING: ■

Calories: 72	Total Carbs: 5 g
Total Fat: 2 g	Dietary Fiber: 1 g
Cholesterol: 4 mg	Protein: 9 g
Sodium: 488 mg	Sugar: 1 g

bruschette

2 cups diced tomatoes
1 cup chopped sweet onions
½ cup chopped fresh parsley
1 teaspoon sea salt
1 teaspoon olive oil

Combine the tomatoes, onions, parsley, salt, and olive oil in a medium bowl and refrigerate until serving. Pile the salsa mixture on the bagel chips and enjoy!

Makes 8 servings; Serving size: ⅓ cup

PER SERVING: ☐

Calories: 22	Total Carbs: 4 g
Total Fat: 1 g	Dietary Fiber: 1 g
Cholesterol: 0 mg	Protein: 1 g
Sodium: 295 mg	Sugar: 0 g

kim's light bagel chips

6 Kim's Light Bagels® (any flavor except blueberry or cinnamon)
Fat-free butter-flavored cooking spray
2 teaspoons garlic salt
1 teaspoon garlic powder

Cut one whole Kim's Light Bagels® in half, so you have two "C" shaped pieces. Each "C" is already presliced. Slice each side again, twice. In the end you will have 8 thin C-shaped bagel chips. Lay chips flat down on a baking sheet, spray lightly with butter-flavored cooking spray. Sprinkle chips with garlic salt and garlic powder. Bake at 350° F for 10 minutes.

Makes 24 servings; Serving size: 2 chips

PER SERVING: ☐

Calories: 28	Total Carbs: 6 g
Total Fat: 0 g	Dietary Fiber: 1 g
Cholesterol: 0 mg	Protein: 1 g
Sodium: 344 mg	Sugar: 0 g

cocktail franks

A family favorite for years . . . now light enough to serve again! With the delicious sauce, you can't even tell the hot dogs are fat-free.

   1 cup yellow mustard
   ⅓ cup honey
   1 cup sugar-free currant or grape jelly
   ½ cup sugar-free orange marmalade
   16 fat-free hot dogs, cut into 8 pieces each

Mix the mustard, honey, jelly, and marmalade in a small saucepan and bring to a boil. Add the hot dog pieces. Serve in a chafing dish with toothpicks.

Makes 32 servings; Serving size: 4 "mini" hot dogs

PER SERVING: ■

Calories: 42	Total Carbs: 8 g
Total Fat: 0 g	Dietary Fiber: 0 g
Cholesterol: 7 mg	Protein: 4 g
Sodium: 331 mg	Sugar: 3 g

filled wontons

Get creative: light cheese and marinara, Asian seasonings, or ham and cheese. Use any filling to make *your* favorite appetizer!

    1 cup diced grilled chicken
    ¼ cup shredded fat-free Cheddar cheese
    ½ teaspoon garlic salt
    ¼ teaspoon freshly ground black pepper
    48 wonton wrappers
    1 cup pizza sauce

Preheat the oven to 350° F. Mince chicken, cheese, garlic salt, and pepper, and mix together in a large bowl. Put 1 tablespoon of the mixture in the center of each wonton wrapper. Fold the wrapper over into a triangle shape, pinching the ends to close, and place on a cookie sheet. Bake for 15 minutes. Serve with a side of sauce for dipping.

Makes 8 servings; Serving size: 6 wontons and 2 tablespoons of sauce

PER SERVING: ■ ■ ■

Calories: 165	Total Carbs: 30 g
Total Fat: 1 g	Dietary Fiber: 1 g
Cholesterol: 11 mg	Protein: 9 g
Sodium: 470 mg	Sugar: 2 g

roasted hummus

When you make your own hummus YOU control the oil, the salt, and the flavor. This flavor mix is delish!

One 15-ounce can chick peas, drained
6 cloves garlic, roasted
1 ounce roasted red peppers, packed in water (reserve
    3 tablespoons water)
¼ teaspoon salt
1 teaspoon olive oil

Put all ingredients into a food processor and pulse until smooth. Enjoy!

Makes 10 servings; Serving size: 2 tablespoons

PER SERVING: ☐

Calories: 31	Total Carbs: 6 g
Total Fat: 1 g	Dietary Fiber: 2 g
Cholesterol: 0 mg	Protein: 2 g
Sodium: 148 mg	Sugar: 0 g

jalapeño poppers

These add a little kick to any party.

2 ounces fat-free cream cheese
½ cup shredded fat-free Cheddar cheese
1 tablespoon fat-free mayonnaise
½ teaspoon salt
1 teaspoon chipotle seasoning
20 small jalapeños
½ cup egg substitute
¾ cup plain bread crumbs
Fat-free cooking spray

Preheat the oven to 350° F. Mix the cheeses, mayonnaise, salt, and chipotle seasoning in a small bowl. Cut the jalapeños lengthwise, leaving the stems on. Discard the seeds. (Use gloves when handling jalapeños and don't touch your eyes!) Divide the cheese mixture among the jalapeño halves. Put the egg substitute in one small bowl and blend the bread crumbs in another. Dip the cheese side of each jalapeño in egg substitute, then in the bread crumbs. Spray the tops of the peppers with fat-free cooking spray to set. Bake for 30 minutes.

Makes 10 servings; Serving size: 4 halves, filled

PER SERVING: ■

Calories: 65	Total Carbs: 8 g
Total Fat: 1 g	Dietary Fiber: 1 g
Cholesterol: 2 mg	Protein: 5 g
Sodium: 300 mg	Sugar: 2 g

layered mexican dip, cold

Make this in a clear glass dish. It looks as good as it tastes.

1⅓ cups fat-free refried beans
½ cup fat-free sour cream
1 cup Mock Guac (page 212)
½ cup chunky salsa, hot or mild to taste
½ cup shredded fat-free Cheddar cheese
5 black olives, thinly sliced
3 tablespoons sliced scallions

Layer the ingredients in the following order: refried beans, sour cream, guacamole, salsa, Cheddar cheese, olives, scallions. Serve cold with low-fat chips or Kim's Light Bagel Chips (page 204).

Makes 10 servings; Serving size: about ⅓ cup

PER SERVING: ■
_____

Calories: 70
Total Fat: 1 g
Cholesterol: 6 mg
Sodium: 349 mg

Total Carbs: 9 g
Dietary Fiber: 2 g
Protein: 5 g
Sugar: 2 g
_____

layered mexican dip, hot

Oh my gosh! This should be its own food group,
it's so good!

    8 ounces fat-free cream cheese
    One 12-ounce can Hormel Turkey Chili
    ½ cup shredded low-fat Cheddar cheese

Preheat the oven to 350° F. Spread the cream cheese in a
small flat baking dish or pie plate. Spread the chili on top.
Sprinkle with the Cheddar cheese. Bake for 15 minutes, or
until bubbly. Let sit for 5 minutes before serving with light
tortilla chips, not factored. That's it. That's all there is to it.
But it is the best dip ever!

Makes 16 servings; Serving size: 3 tablespoons

PER SERVING: ■

Calories: 75	Total Carbs: 6 g
Total Fat: 1 g	Dietary Fiber: 1 g
Cholesterol: 13 mg	Protein: 10 g
Sodium: 438 mg	Sugar: 2 g

mini-blts

When you want the flavor of a BLT without all the carbs.

1 pound Campari tomatoes
3 cups chopped iceberg lettuce
3 tablespoons real bacon bits (like Hormel)
½ teaspoon celery salt
1 teaspoon salt
½ cup fat-free mayonnaise

Cut the tomatoes in half horizontally and scoop out the seeds and flesh in the middle, leaving the flesh and skin on the outer edge. Mix the lettuce, bacon bits, celery salt, salt, and mayonnaise. Fill the tomato halves with the lettuce and bacon mixture and serve.

Makes 12 servings; Serving size: 2 halves, filled

PER SERVING: ☐
___

Calories: 13	Total Carbs: 2 g
Total Fat: 0 g	Dietary Fiber: 0 g
Cholesterol: 1 mg	Protein: 1 g
Sodium: 200 mg	Sugar: 0 g
___

For non-T (tomato) lovers, substitute hard-boiled egg whites for the tomatoes. Simply cut a hard-boiled egg in half and discard the yolk. Fill the egg whites with the lettuce mixture.

mock guac

Avocado is high in fat and calories. Yes, it's a healthy fat, but if you're on a diet, ½ cup of guacamole has 187 calories and 18 grams of fat! Yowza! Our Mock Guac uses peas as a base—the perfect high-fiber substitute. Try it and don't tell anyone. They won't even know!

2 cups frozen peas
1½ cups fat-free sour cream
½ cup reduced fat sour cream
3 tablespoons ripe avocado
1 tablespoon lime juice
3 garlic cloves
1 tablespoon ground cumin
1 teaspoon garlic salt
1 teaspoon hot sauce
1 large tomato, chopped small
1 cup onion, diced

Microwave the frozen peas in a covered bowl for 2 minutes. Drain VERY WELL and lay on a paper towel to absorb all the water. You can even squeeze to make sure they're very dry. In a food processor, puree the peas, sour cream, avocado, lime juice, cloves, cumin, garlic salt, and hot sauce. Fold in the chopped tomatoes (be sure they are drained as much as possible) and onions. Chill for at least 1 hour before serving. Yum!

Makes 16 servings; Serving size: ¼ cup

PER SERVING: ■

Calories: 58	Total Carbs: 7 g
Total Fat: 2 g	Dietary Fiber: 2 g
Cholesterol: 7 mg	Protein: 3 g
Sodium: 72 mg	Sugar: 3 g

oysters parmesan

An oyster recipe that even the non–seafood lover will love! Well, maybe not all of them.

- ¼ cup 98 percent fat-free chicken broth
- 2 teaspoons olive oil
- ⅔ cup bread crumbs
- 2 teaspoons minced garlic
- ¼ cup minced fresh parsley
- ½ cup grated reduced-fat Parmesan cheese
- 48 fresh oysters

Preheat the oven to 400° F. Heat the broth and olive oil in a skillet over medium heat. Add the bread crumbs and garlic, stirring for approximately 3 minutes. Add the parsley and Parmesan cheese. Shuck the oysters, reserving the shells. Clean the shells and lay 48 of them on a cookie sheet on their backs. In a small bowl, combine the oysters and the bread-crumb mixture. Spoon an oyster into each half shell, heavily surrounded by the bread-crumb mixture. Bake for 10 minutes. Serve warm in the shell. You can substitute clams if desired.

Makes 16 servings; Serving size: 3 oysters

PER SERVING: ■■

Calories: 73	Total Carbs: 8 g
Total Fat: 3 g	Dietary Fiber: 0 g
Cholesterol: 19 mg	Protein: 4 g
Sodium: 205 mg	Sugar: 0 g

LOW-CARB OPTION: Substitute ⅔ cup real bacon bits for the bread crumbs and shredded low-fat mozzarella cheese for the Parmesan cheese.

party shrimp dip

A recipe everyone at your next party will be asking for.

Two 4-ounce cans baby shrimp
One 10¾-ounce can fat-free cream of mushroom soup
8 ounces fat-free cream cheese
16 ounces fat-free mayonnaise
1 small bunch scallions, chopped
1 envelope Knox gelatin
Freshly ground black pepper

Drain 1 of the cans of shrimp. Mix the soup and cream cheese in a saucepan and heat until warm. Remove from the heat and mix in both cans of shrimp, the mayonnaise, and scallions until well blended. Dilute the gelatin with 1 tablespoon cold water and then stir into the dip. Add pepper to taste. Pour the dip into a mold or the final serving container and chill in the fridge for several hours or overnight. It tastes delicious and is very light—yet thick and creamy. I always leave a few baby shrimp and a green onion on top as a garnish. Serve with your favorite light chips or crackers (not included in nutrition info.).

Makes 32 servings; Serving size: ¼ cup

PER SERVING: ■

Calories: 34	Total Carbs: 4 g
Total Fat: 1 g	Dietary Fiber: 1 g
Cholesterol: 14 mg	Protein: 3 g
Sodium: 287 mg	Sugar: 2 g

snack mix

We've worked really hard at getting this as light as possible.
After all, it's important to have a great snack mix that fits
your diet plan, isn't it?!

4 cups Rice Chex cereal

2 cups Corn Chex cereal

3 cups puffed rice cereal

½ cup Fiber One cereal

3 ounces small pretzel sticks

16 Kim's Light Bagel Chips* (see page 204)

Fat-free butter-flavored cooking spray

½ cup Worcestershire sauce

2 teaspoons seasoned salt

¾ teaspoon garlic powder

Preheat the oven to 300° F. Mix the cereals, pretzel sticks,
and bagel chips in a deep baking pan. Carefully toss with fat-
free butter-flavored cooking spray while slowly sprinkling in
the Worcestershire, seasoned salt, and garlic powder, one by
one. Bake for 15 to 20 minutes, turning halfway through.
The mix should be dry, but not burned. Let cool and store in
an airtight container.

Makes 20 servings; Serving size: ⅔ cup

* Factored using 2 Kim's Light Bagel Chips (see page 204)

PER SERVING: ■

Calories: 79	Total Carbs: 17 g
Total Fat: 0 g	Dietary Fiber: 1 g
Cholesterol: 0 mg	Protein: 2 g
Sodium: 461 mg	Sugar: 2 g

stuffed mushrooms

4 ounces seasoned stuffing mix

50 medium white mushrooms, about 2 pounds

¼ cup finely chopped scallions

¼ cup finely chopped red bell pepper

½ teaspoon garlic salt

2 teaspoons Brummel & Brown® Buttery Spread

1 tablespoon fat-free Parmesan cheese

2 tablespoons shredded fat-free Cheddar cheese

Preheat the broiler. Prepare the stuffing mix, omitting the margarine. Clean the mushroom caps and remove the stems. Sauté the scallions, bell pepper, and garlic salt in the Brummel & Brown and ¼ cup water for approximately 7 minutes, until tender. Add the stuffing and combine. Stuff the mushrooms and top with the cheeses. Broil for 3 to 5 minutes.

Makes 10 servings; Serving size: 5 mushrooms

PER SERVING: ■

Calories: 95	Total Carbs: 12 g
Total Fat: 1 g	Dietary Fiber: 2 g
Cholesterol: 1 mg	Protein: 5 g
Sodium: 225 mg	Sugar: 3 g

LOW-CARB OPTION: Substitute cooked ground sausage for the stuffing mix. Drops carbs to 3 grams net per serving.

wasabi chick peas

This crunchy, light, and spicy snack is great for the road, the office, or the movie theater.

> Two 15-ounce cans chick peas, drained and rinsed
> 1 teaspoon sea salt, to taste
> 3 tablespoons wasabi powder*
> Olive oil cooking spray

In a large zip-top bag, add the chick peas, the salt, and wasabi powder. Shake until all chick peas are coated completely. Lay flat on a baking sheet. Bake at 400° F for 40 minutes, shaking the tray often. Allow to cool completely and serve as a nut or take it on the road as a snack.

* If you like more of a kick, add more wasabi.

Makes 4 servings; Serving size: ¼ cup

PER SERVING: ■

Calories: 100	Total Carbs: 10 g
Total Fat: 2 g	Dietary Fiber: 3 g
Cholesterol: 0 mg	Protein: 3 g
Sodium: 471 mg	Sugar: 0 g

salads

chop chop salad

The great thing about chopped salads are that the flavors of the vegetables and fruits blend together in a delightful way before you even start to chew. I did a TV shoot at the Rock Center Café in New York City and fell in love with their chopped salad. This is my rendition.

SALAD:

½ cup chopped Napa cabbage
3 cups chopped romaine lettuce
½ cup chopped red onion
¼ cup chopped scallions
1 cup chopped celery
½ cup chopped red bell pepper
1 apple, chopped
Fresh parsley sprigs

ASIAN DRESSING:

3 garlic cloves, minced
2 tablespoons minced fresh ginger
1 tablespoon sesame oil
½ cup rice vinegar
¼ cup soy sauce
2 teaspoons honey

SALAD: Make sure the vegetables are completely dry before chopping—they release moisture as you chop, and you don't want a soggy salad. Put the apple and all of the vegetables except the parsley in a large bowl and chop until the pieces are very small, but not minced. You can purchase Toss & Chop scissors designed for this purpose at most kitchen supply stores, or you can hand-chop the vegetables on a wooden board.

To plate the salad, fill a small bowl with approximately 1¼ cups of the salad, packing it slightly, and then turn the bowl upside down on a small plate. The damp vegetables should hold their dome shape. Garnish with a sprig of parsley and drizzle with 2 tablespoons Asian Dressing. You can add chicken or shrimp to make this salad a main course.

ASIAN DRESSING: Combine the garlic, ginger, sesame oil, vinegar, soy sauce, honey, and 3 tablespoons water in a 1-pint glass jar. Cover tightly and shake well. Remove the lid and heat the dressing in a microwave oven for approximately 1 minute, or until the dressing heats enough to melt the honey. Put the lid back on and shake well before serving. Store in the refrigerator for up to 2 weeks.

Makes 6 servings; Serving size: 1 cup

PER SERVING: ■

Calories: 75	Total Carbs: 13 g
Total Fat: 2 g	Dietary Fiber: 2 g
Cholesterol: 0 mg	Protein: 2 g
Sodium: 622 mg	Sugar: 4 g

three-bean salad

I never liked bean salads growing up. A three-bean salad was served at our beans-and-hot-dogs suppers on steamy summer evenings in Maine, and I always passed it by. I'm not a big canned-bean lover. This one's different. Trust me. If I had to pick, I think this would be my favorite recipe in the book. It's that good! Try it.

2 tablespoons white wine vinegar
2 tablespoons red wine vinegar
½ cup chopped fresh basil
1½ teaspoons olive oil
Salt and freshly ground black pepper, to taste
¾ cup red kidney beans, drained and rinsed
¾ cup cannellini beans, drained and rinsed
4 cups sliced fresh green beans, snapped and steamed slightly
½ cup sliced scallions

Combine the vinegars, basil, and olive oil in a small bowl and season to taste with salt and pepper. Combine the beans and scallions in a large bowl and pour the dressing over them. Toss gently and refrigerate before serving.

Makes 8 servings; Serving size: ¾ cup

PER SERVING: ■

Calories: 68	Total Carbs: 12 g
Total Fat: 1 g	Dietary Fiber: 5 g
Cholesterol: 0 mg	Protein: 4 g
Sodium: 707 mg	Sugar: 0 g

cool cucumber salad

Cool. Crisp. Delightful.

    1 English cucumber, scored lengthwise with a fork
      and thinly sliced (about 4 cups)
    ½ cup red or sweet onion, thinly sliced
    1 teaspoon olive oil
    2 tablespoons cider vinegar
    2 teaspoons sugar substitute
    1 teaspoon sea salt
    ½ teaspoon freshly ground black pepper

Combine the cucumber and onion slices in a medium bowl.
Combine the remaining ingredients in a small bowl. Add the
dressing to the cucumber and onion slices and toss well.
Cover and refrigerate for up to 2 hours before serving.

Makes 4 servings; Serving size: about 1 cup

PER SERVING: ☐

Calories: 30	Total Carbs: 5 g
Total Fat: 1 g	Dietary Fiber: 1 g
Cholesterol: 0 mg	Protein: 1 g
Sodium: 585 mg	Sugar: 2 g

green whipped salad

A sweet side dish that's great to pull out again when it's time for dessert.

> One 1-ounce package fat-free, sugar-free instant pistachio pudding mix
> One 16-ounce can crushed pineapple, drained
> 8 ounces fat-free whipped topping

Mix all of the ingredients together. Refrigerate for 2 to 3 hours before serving.

Makes 12 servings; Serving size: ½ cup

PER SERVING: ■

Calories: 63	Total Carbs: 14 g
Total Fat: 0 g	Dietary Fiber: 0 g
Cholesterol: 0 mg	Protein: 0 g
Sodium: 120 mg	Sugar: 6 g

light waldorf salad

The original recipe, created by Oscar Tschirky, the maitre d'hotel of the Waldorf-Astoria Hotel in New York City, called for only celery, apples, and mayonnaise. It soon became a staple in most hotel dining rooms. Later walnuts were added, and other variations have since emerged. Now, welcome our Light Waldorf Salad.

2¾ cups chopped apples
1 cup diced celery
¼ cup raisins
7 walnut halves, coarsely chopped
7 tablespoons fat-free mayonnaise
2 tablespoons sugar substitute
1 teaspoon lemon juice

Combine the apples, celery, raisins, and walnuts in a large bowl. Mix the mayonnaise, sugar substitute, and lemon juice in a small bowl until well blended. Add the dressing to the fruit mixture and toss.

Makes 6 servings; Serving size: ⅔ cup

PER SERVING: ■

Calories: 89	Total Carbs: 18 g
Total Fat: 2 g	Dietary Fiber: 3 g
Cholesterol: 2 mg	Protein: 1 g
Sodium: 158 mg	Sugar: 1 g

new potato salad

I first tasted this recipe at a picnic when I was still very heavy. At the time I would *never* eat anything made with light or fat-free mayonnaise. I tried this potato salad and liked it so much that I continued to go back for more until it was nearly gone. I asked for the recipe and to my amazement was told it was fat free! The fresh dill makes it!

1¾ pounds new red potatoes
½ cup fat-free mayonnaise
½ cup fat-free plain yogurt
1 teaspoon salt
¾ cup sliced scallions, the white part only
½ cup chopped fresh dill

Boil the potatoes, leaving the skins on, until cooked but not overdone. Cool and cut carefully into quarters. In a large bowl, blend the mayonnaise, yogurt, and salt, and toss gently with the potatoes, scallions, and dill. Chill until ready to serve.

Makes 8 servings; Serving size: ½ cup

PER SERVING: ■

Calories: 72	Total Carbs: 16 g
Total Fat: 0 g	Dietary Fiber: 2 g
Cholesterol: 0 mg	Protein: 2 g
Sodium: 443 mg	Sugar: 3 g

seven-layer salad

I never thought I'd eat this summer favorite salad again, but with the right choice of ingredients, we've made it just as delicious, beautiful to look at . . . and light!

6 cups romaine lettuce, shredded
3 large carrots, sliced
1 can sliced water chestnuts
One 10-ounce bag of frozen baby peas, defrosted
1 cup fat-free shredded Cheddar cheese
½ cup Smart Beat® Mayonnaise*
½ cup Oscar Mayer® precooked bacon, crumbled

In a large clear bowl, fill the bottom with shredded lettuce. Layer sliced carrots next. Drain the water chestnuts and layer them on top of the carrots. Layer the defrosted peas over the water chestnuts. Sprinkle the Cheddar cheese over the top of the water chestnuts. Spread the *Smart Beat Mayonnaise over the top of the entire mixture and sprinkle crumbled bacon pieces over it.

You should be able to clearly see the layers through the side of the clear bowl. Beautiful and yummy! Serve immediately.

Makes 8 servings; Serving size: 1¼ cups

PER SERVING: ■

Calories: 94	Total Carbs: 13 g
Total Fat: 1 g	Dietary Fiber: 3 g
Cholesterol: 6 mg	Protein: 8 g
Sodium: 377 mg	Sugar: 4 g

summer salsa

Make it up ahead of time. Makes a great dip or use it on top of your favorite greens for a refreshing summer salad.

One 11-ounce can white corn, drained, not rinsed
One 15.5-ounce can black beans, drained, not rinsed
1 cup scallions, chopped
½ cup fat-free Italian dressing
½ cup red bell pepper, finely diced
½ cup yellow bell pepper, finely diced
½ cup green bell pepper, finely diced

Combine all ingredients and refrigerate until ready to serve. Serve with Kim's Light Bagel Chips (see page 204; not factored in nutrition info.).

Makes 10 servings; Serving size: ⅓ cup

PER SERVING: ■
_____

Calories: 105
Total Fat: 0 g
Cholesterol: 0 mg
Sodium: 230 mg

Total Carbs: 21 g
Dietary Fiber: 3 g
Protein: 4 g
Sugar: 3 g
_____

tomato-mozzarella salad

A lightened-up version of a yummy recipe from Bertucci's, one of my favorite Italian restaurants, where I used to waitress.

2 teaspoons olive oil
1 teaspoon lemon juice, optional
1 teaspoon sea salt
½ cup chopped fresh basil
3 garlic cloves, minced
5 cups ripe plum tomatoes, cut into eighths
1½ cups small part-skim mozzarella cheese balls
½ cup sliced sweet onion, rings separated

Mix the olive oil, lemon juice, salt, basil, and garlic in a small bowl. Let the mixture sit for an hour or longer; overnight is best to mix the flavors. Toss with the tomatoes, mozzarella cheese balls, and onion. Chill for 30 minutes and serve.

Makes 8 servings; Serving size: ¾ cup

PER SERVING: ■■

Calories: 121	Total Carbs: 10 g
Total Fat: 6 g	Dietary Fiber: 3 g
Cholesterol: 16 mg	Protein: 9 g
Sodium: 435 mg	Sugar: 0 g

side dishes

broccoli crunch

This great side dish has been used by many moms to get kids to eat their broccoli when they won't look at it plain. And yes, you can use it for husbands, too.

One 10¾-ounce can 98-percent fat-free cheesy broccoli soup
¼ cup fat-free mayonnaise
Four 10-ounce packages frozen chopped broccoli, thawed
20 reduced-fat Ritz crackers
Fat-free butter-flavored cooking spray

Preheat the oven to 350° F. Mix the soup and mayonnaise in a bowl. Add the broccoli and toss lightly to coat. Pour the mixture into a casserole dish. Crush the crackers and sprinkle on top of the casserole. Spray lightly with fat-free cooking spray to moisten the crackers slightly. Bake for 20 minutes, or until heated through.

Makes 8 servings; Serving size: ¾ cup

PER SERVING: ■

Calories: 71	Total Carbs: 12 g
Total Fat: 1 g	Dietary Fiber: 5 g
Cholesterol: 1 mg	Protein: 5 g
Sodium: 283 mg	Sugar: 2 g

cheesy french fry casserole

A kid favorite. An adult favorite, too.

6 cups frozen shredded hash brown potatoes
One 10.75-ounce can of 98-percent fat-free cream of chicken soup
4 ounces fat-free sour cream
3 ounces fat-free shredded cheddar cheese
½ cup onion, finely diced
¼ teaspoon cayenne pepper
1 teaspoon salt
½ teaspoon pepper

Preheat oven to 375° F. Combine all ingredients in a bowl. Spray a baking dish with fat-free cooking spray. Transfer mixture to the baking dish. Bake about 1 hour or until bubbly and golden on top. Brown under broiler, if desired.

Makes 4 servings; Serving size: ¼ cup

PER SERVING: ■

Calories: 89	Total Carbs: 15 g
Total Fat: 1 g	Dietary Fiber: 2 g
Cholesterol: 5 mg	Protein: 5 g
Sodium: 516 mg	Sugar: 2 g

dirty potatoes

Not really dirty of course, but the skins add to that old-fashioned look. A scrumptious, hearty side dish.

    6 cups diced unpeeled potatoes
    4 tablespoons fat-free cream cheese
    4 tablespoons fat-free half-and-half
    1 tablespoon fat-free spray butter
    2 teaspoons crushed garlic
    2 teaspoons garlic salt

Place the potatoes in a large pot, cover with water, and boil approximately 15 minutes, or until tender. Drain. Using an electric mixer or a potato masher, mix in the remaining ingredients. Goes great with No-Guilt Gravy (page 233)!

Makes 12 servings; Serving size: ½ cup

PER SERVING: ■
_____

Calories: 71   Total Carbs: 14 g
Total Fat: 0 g   Dietary Fiber: 2 g
Cholesterol: 2 mg   Protein: 3 g
Sodium: 69 mg   Sugar: 1 g
_____

feta & olives

Premade Feta and Olives is usually found at the deli counter in the supermarkets—swimming in oil! Now you can make your own with all the flavor and very little fat.

    6 ounces small black olives*
    6 ounces green olives*
    8 ounces fat-free feta cheese
    1 tablespoon olive oil

*Reserve 2 tablespoons of each flavor of olive juices and mix with olive oil. Cube the feta and mix all the ingredients. Lightly toss to evenly disperse the olive-oil mixture. Serve chilled.

Makes 16 servings; Serving size: ¼ cup

PER SERVING: ■

Calories: 55	Total Carbs: 1 g
Total Fat: 2 g	Dietary Fiber: 1 g
Cholesterol: 0 mg	Protein: 0 g
Sodium: 249 mg	Sugar: 0 g

light pesto

Use with light pasta, baked potatoes, or as a spread.

7 walnut halves
2½ cups fresh basil leaves, packed
3 garlic cloves
2 tablespoons extra-virgin olive oil
6 tablespoons water
3½ tablespoons fat-free Parmesan cheese
1 teaspoon sea salt
Dash of freshly ground black pepper

Pulse the walnuts a few times in the bowl of a food processor and then add the basil leaves. Pulse a few more times. Add the garlic and pulse a few more times. Add the olive oil and 6 tablespoons water and leave the food processor on for a minute or two. Stop to scrape down the sides with a rubber spatula. Add the Parmesan cheese and pulse again until blended. Add the salt and pepper. Pulse one more time.

Makes 10 servings; Serving size: 2 tablespoons

PER SERVING: ■
_____

Calories: 58
Total Fat: 5 g
Cholesterol: 5 mg
Sodium: 541 mg

Total Carbs: 3 g
Dietary Fiber: 1 g
Protein: 2 g
Sugar: 0 g
_____

no-guilt gravy

Every holiday I was in charge of making the gravy. I, of course, used all the fat from the bird. It was very delicious, but so fattening! I substituted this for my gravy the first Thanksgiving after I began Weight Watchers. To my amazement, no one knew the difference! Now you can pour on the gravy without worrying about all the fat! You gotta love those 98-percent fat-free Campbell's soups!

Two 10¾-ounce cans 98-percent fat-free cream of chicken soup
2 ounces reduced-fat chicken broth
¼ teaspoon Gravy Master seasoning
½ teaspoon garlic powder
1 teaspoon poultry seasoning
½ teaspoon freshly ground black pepper
2 tablespoons nonfat milk
2 teaspoons cornstarch

Mix the soup, broth, gravy seasoning, garlic powder, poultry seasoning, and pepper in a medium saucepan. Heat and simmer for 7 minutes. Mix the milk and cornstarch in a small bowl. Bring the gravy mixture to a boil and gradually stir in the milk mixture. Continue to cook, stirring constantly, for 1 minute or until thickened. Be careful not to let the bottom scorch.

Makes 16 servings; Serving size: ¼ cup

PER SERVING: ☐

Calories: 29	Total Carbs: 4 g
Total Fat: 1 g	Dietary Fiber: 1 g
Cholesterol: 4 mg	Protein: 1 g
Sodium: 229 mg	Sugar: 0 g

recipes

potatoes au gratin

A classic side dish and favorite of my oldest son, Adam.

Fat-free cooking spray
1 teaspoon Brummel & Brown® Buttery Spread
1 medium onion, thinly sliced
2 tablespoons all-purpose flour
2 cups nonfat milk
6 cups potatoes, thinly sliced
1 cup shredded fat-free Cheddar cheese
1 teaspoon salt
¼ teaspoon freshly ground black pepper

Preheat the oven to 375° F. Spray a large baking dish with fat-free cooking spray. Melt the Brummel & Brown in a large nonstick pot. Add the onion and sauté, stirring occasionally until golden brown. Add the flour and milk, stirring slowly. Add the potatoes and bring to a boil. Add ¾ cup of the cheese and season with salt and pepper.

Pour the mixture into the baking dish. Cover and bake for 30 to 45 minutes, until the potatoes are soft. Keep an eye on this; if you are using a more shallow dish, it will take less time. Uncover and bake for another 20 minutes. Sprinkle the remaining cheese over the dish. Broil for 1 to 2 minutes, or until the cheese is golden brown. Cool for about 5 minutes before dividing into 9 pieces.

Makes 9 servings; Serving size: about ⅔ cup

PER SERVING: ■■

Calories: 128	Total Carbs: 24 g
Total Fat: 0 g	Dietary Fiber: 3 g
Cholesterol: 3 mg	Protein: 8 g
Sodium: 418 mg	Sugar: 4 g

smashed cauliflower

A great way to fill up your plate at the holidays, but use it all year long. Beware: Many restaurant versions are very high in fat. This one just tastes that way.

1 large head cauliflower
2 cloves garlic, peeled and chopped
1 tablespoon fat-free half-and-half
Salt and freshly ground black pepper
Grated fat-free Parmesan cheese, optional (not factored)

Steam or boil the whole head of cauliflower in a large pot just until tender. Drain *very* well. Add the remaining ingredients and beat for several minutes with an electric mixer. Top with fat-free Parmesan cheese, if desired (not included in nutrition info.).

Makes 4 servings; Serving size: 1 cup

PER SERVING: ☐

Calories: 57	Total Carbs: 12 g
Total Fat: 0 g	Dietary Fiber: 5 g
Cholesterol: 0 mg	Protein: 4 g
Sodium: 107 mg	Sugar: 0 g

spinach fillo

Another great recipe from my favorite aunt. I love you, Tina!

Fat-free cooking spray
8 sheets fillo dough
6 ounces fat-free feta cheese, crumbled
Three 10-ounce packages frozen spinach, thawed and
   well drained
1 cup egg substitute
1 tablespoon salt

Preheat the oven to 350° F. Spray a 9 × 13-inch baking dish
lightly with fat-free cooking spray for 3 seconds and lay
2 sheets of fillo in the dish. Spray for 2 seconds and lay
another sheet of fillo in the dish. Repeat two more times (for
a total of 5 sheets of fillo). Mix the remaining ingredients and
pour on top of the fillo. Finish with 3 sheets of fillo and spray
for 2 seconds. Bake for 30 minutes.

Makes 10 servings; Serving size: ¹⁄₁₂ of recipe

PER SERVING: ■

Calories: 78	Total Carbs: 11 g
Total Fat: 1 g	Dietary Fiber: 2 g
Cholesterol: 0 mg	Protein: 8 g
Sodium: 1,080 mg	Sugar: 0 g

twice-baked potatoes

Twice-baked means twice as good, but not twice as fattening.

  4 medium baking potatoes
  ¼ cup fat-free sour cream
  ¼ cup nonfat milk
  2 slices Oscar Mayer® fully-cooked bacon, crumbled
  ½ cup shredded fat-free Cheddar cheese
  ½ cup sliced scallions
  2 teaspoons salt
  1 teaspoon freshly ground black pepper

Preheat the oven to 350° F. Wrap the potatoes in aluminum foil and bake for 45 minutes until soft *or* cook for 15 minutes (without foil) in a microwave oven. Cut the potatoes completely in half lengthwise. Scoop out the center of each potato, leaving a shell ⅛ inch thick all the way around, and reserve the skins. Mash the potatoes with the remaining ingredients until creamy. Fill each potato skin with ⅛ of the filling mixture, using a pastry bag if desired. Bake again for 15 minutes, or until the tops are slightly brown.

Makes 8 servings; Serving size: ½ of loaded potato

PER SERVING: ■

Calories: 80	Total Carbs: 15 g
Total Fat: 1 g	Dietary Fiber: 1 g
Cholesterol: 32 mg	Protein: 4 g
Sodium: 668 mg	Sugar: 1 g

baked beans

1 medium onion, chopped

½ cup pineapple, chopped

5 slices precooked bacon, chopped

Two 15-ounce cans red kidney beans, 1 drained

One 15-ounce can navy beans, drained

¼ cup sugar-free maple syrup

½ cup ketchup

1 teaspoon mustard

1 teaspoon onion powder

Sauté the onions, pineapple, and bacon, until the onions start to become translucent. Pour all ingredients into an oven-safe crock and cover. Bake for 45 minutes at 350°F. Uncover and bake another 15 minutes. Allow to cool slightly and serve.

Makes 12 servings; Serving size: ½ cup

PER SERVING: ■

Calories: 106	Total Carbs: 19 g
Total Fat: 1 g	Dietary Fiber: 6 g
Cholesterol: 3 mg	Protein: 7 g
Sodium: 464 mg	Sugar: 3 g

soups

bean chili

When I first saw this recipe written on the easel at my Weight Watchers meeting, I thought it sounded gross and didn't even copy it down, but my girlfriend Cathy did. She made it later that week, and we've both loved it ever since.

I put a head of shredded lettuce on a plate and pour a cup of Bean Chili over it. Then I top it all with a little shredded light Cheddar cheese and a few homemade fat-free taco chips. It's a whole lot of food for very few calories.

One 15-ounce can black beans
One 15-ounce can kidney beans
One 15-ounce can cannellini beans
One 15-ounce can black-eyed peas
Two 15-ounce cans diced tomatoes, with or without green chiles
1 package taco seasoning
1 package fat-free ranch dip mix (I use Hidden Valley)
3 cups diced green bell pepper
3 cups diced celery

Do not drain the beans! Mix all of the ingredients in a large pot and simmer until the veggies are just tender, about 10 minutes. Try it. You'll like it.

Makes 18 servings; Serving size: 1 cup

PER SERVING: ■

Calories: 110	Total Carbs: 19 g
Total Fat: 0 g	Dietary Fiber: 7 g
Cholesterol: 0 mg	Protein: 7 g
Sodium: 331 mg	Sugar: 2 g

cream of broccoli soup

This is the recipe referred to in my success story on the weightwatchers.com Web site.

Two 10-ounce packages frozen chopped broccoli, thawed
1 large onion, chopped
5 cups fat-free chicken broth
1½ teaspoons salt
1½ teaspoons freshly ground black pepper
2 tablespoons fat-free half-and-half

Put 1½ packages of broccoli and the onion, broth, and salt into a large pot. Bring to a boil and simmer until the broccoli is tender, about 10 minutes. Using a blender, purée the contents, a little at a time. Pour the puréed soup back into the large pot and add the rest of the broccoli for a chunky soup. Add the pepper and half-and-half. Heat and serve. If you like the soup thicker, start with all of the broccoli. If you like it thinner, start with less of the broccoli.

Makes 6 servings; Serving size: 1 cup

PER SERVING: ☐

Calories: 40	Total Carbs: 7 g
Total Fat: 1 g	Dietary Fiber: 3 g
Cholesterol: 0 mg	Protein: 4 g
Sodium: 627 mg	Sugar: 2 g

downeast chowdah

Go to Maine. Take a ferry to Peaks Island, knock on my parents' front door, and ask my mom to make this for you. No
one makes it like she does. An entire filling meal in a bowl.
(Uh, just kidding about going to my parents' house!)

Fat-free cooking spray
1 large onion, chopped
4 cups water
¾ teaspoon dried thyme
2 teaspoons dried parsley
2 cups chopped celery
2¾ cups diced potatoes
1 tablespoon salt
Freshly ground black pepper
1¼ pounds fresh cod fillets (or your favorite white fish)
¾ cup fat-free half-and-half

Spray a large saucepan with fat-free cooking spray for
5 seconds. Add the onion and lightly toss over medium heat
for 2 minutes. Add 4 cups water and the thyme, parsley,
celery, potatoes, salt, and pepper to taste. Cover and cook
for 10 minutes over medium heat. Lay the cod fillets on top of
the chowder. Cover and let steam (still on medium heat) until
the fish is cooked, about 10 minutes. Add the half-and-half.
Stir gently to break up the fish slightly. Do not boil after adding
the half-and-half.

Makes 12 servings; Serving size: 1 cup

PER SERVING: ■■

Calories: 140	Total Carbs: 14 g
Total Fat: 1 g	Dietary Fiber: 2 g
Cholesterol: 40 mg	Protein: 18 g
Sodium: 993 mg	Sugar: 2 g

hamburger soup

A recipe from Shirl Jacobsen, a dear friend (and exercise buddy) since I was sixteen. She recently married a really nice guy named Bob at the lovely young age of eighty-six! Way to go, Shirl—see what exercise will do for you!

- ¾ pound 93-percent fat-free ground beef
- 2 cups canned tomatoes
- 3 cups diced carrots
- 2 cups diced celery
- 1 onion, diced
- 1 tablespoon salt
- ¼ teaspoon freshly ground black pepper
- ¼ cup uncooked brown rice
- 3 beef bouillon cubes
- 8 cups water

Put all of the ingredients into a large pot. Add 8 cups water, bring to a boil, and stir to break up the meat. Reduce the heat and simmer for 45 minutes. (Before there was 93-percent lean meat, we used to let the soup sit in the refrigerator overnight and spoon the fat off the top in the morning before eating. Now it makes so little fat, this step isn't necessary.)

Makes 12 servings; Serving size: 1 cup

PER SERVING: ■

Calories: 75	Total Carbs: 7 g
Total Fat: 2 g	Dietary Fiber: 2 g
Cholesterol: 16 mg	Protein: 7 g
Sodium: 909 mg	Sugar: 3 g

italian escarole soup

I had never cooked with escarole before making this soup.
It's light and lovely.

1 head escarole
6 cups 98-percent fat-free chicken broth
2 large links chicken sausage, sliced
2 chicken bouillon cubes
1 teaspoon dried oregano
1 teaspoon dried basil
3 garlic cloves, chopped
Salt to taste

Wash the escarole well and cut into salad-size bites. Put the
escarole, broth, sausage, bouillon, oregano, basil, and garlic
in a large pot and bring to a boil. Reduce the heat to medium-
low and simmer for 30 minutes. Add salt to taste. You can
top this with fat-free Parmesan cheese, if desired (not
included in nutritional info).

Makes 6 servings; Serving size: 1 cup

PER SERVING:

Calories: 63	Total Carbs: 2 g
Total Fat: 2 g	Dietary Fiber: 1 g
Cholesterol: 23 mg	Protein: 8 g
Sodium: 1,299 mg	Sugar: 0 g

wild rice soup

This is a Minnesota dish that is perfect for a cold winter day and will leave everyone satisfied. Thanks, Sissy!

2 cups wild rice, cooked (can use brown)
Spray butter, 5 sprays
¼ cup onion, minced
2 tablespoons cornstarch
½ teaspoon salt
2 tablespoons fresh parsley, chopped
2 teaspoons fresh thyme, chopped
4 cups vegetable broth
1 cup carrots, finely chopped
1 cup celery, finely chopped
3 tablespoons almonds, finely chopped
2 tablespoons Sherry cooking wine
½ cup fat-free half & half
salt and pepper to taste

Cook the rice and set aside until ready to add.

Spray the spray butter in a pan and sauté the onions until tender. Add cornstarch, salt, parsley, thyme, and vegetable broth. Bring to a boil and cook for 1 minute. Stir in the remaining ingredients except the half & half. Simmer for 5 minutes, then add the half & half. This is delicious piping hot with homemade bread and marinated veggies.

Note that this is a thick soup and it will thicken as it sits. Also, be sure you make the rice according to the package. For best results, do not use instant rice. Chicken broth can be switched out for the vegetable broth.

Makes 6 servings; Serving size: 1 cup

PER SERVING: ■ ■

Calories: 126	Total Carbs: 22 g
Total Fat: 2 g	Dietary Fiber: 2 g
Cholesterol: 1 mg	Protein: 4 g
Sodium: 889 mg	Sugar: 4 g

entrées

american chop suey

Comfort food at its best!

2 cups whole-wheat macaroni, cooked
Fat-free cooking spray
1 cup chopped onion
1 cup chopped green bell pepper
12 ounces lean ground turkey
3 cups diced tomatoes
4 slices fat-free American cheese
1 tablespoon soy sauce
1 teaspoon chili powder
1 teaspoon salt

Lightly spray a nonstick frying pan with fat-free cooking spray and add the onion and bell pepper. Add the turkey and fry over low-medium heat until cooked, stirring frequently. Add the tomatoes, cheese, soy sauce, chili powder, salt, and macaroni. Stir until blended. Simmer for 10 minutes.

Makes 10 servings; Serving size: 1 cup

PER SERVING: ■■

Calories: 127	Total Carbs: 16 g
Total Fat: 3 g	Dietary Fiber: 2 g
Cholesterol: 25 mg	Protein: 11 g
Sodium: 554 mg	Sugar: 4 g

cheese tortellini

Who doesn't like cheese tortellini? But at 320 calories per cup, it can be really hard to fit in to a healthy meal plan. Move over Chef Boyardee. This recipe will kick your can!

15 ounces fat-free ricotta cheese
2 ounces Egg Beaters®
1 tablespoon parsley flakes
60 wonton wrappers

Blend Egg Beaters® into ricotta cheese along with parsley flakes. On each wonton, place 1½ teaspoon of cheese mixture in the center of the wrapper. Fold over to make a triangle. Seal it by dipping your finger in water and moistening the edges of the wrapper. After it is a triangle, attach the two points, and fold over the top to form a tortellini. Place in boiling water and boil for 4 minutes. Remove from the water and top with your favorite low-calorie red or white sauce (not included in nutritional information).

Makes 10 servings; Serving size: 6 tortellinis

PER SERVING: ■ ■ ■

Calories: 165	Total Carbs: 29 g
Total Fat: 1 g	Dietary Fiber: 1 g
Cholesterol: 4 mg	Protein: 10 g
Sodium: 304 mg	Sugar: 2 g

cheesy chicken enchiladas

Oh my gosh! Who cares whether the chicken or the egg came first! I'm just glad there's chicken in this fantastic entrée!

1½ cups (22 ounces) cooked, shredded chicken breast
5 cups fresh baby spinach
¼ cup sliced scallions, plus more for garnish
1½ cups fat-free sour cream
¼ cup nonfat plain yogurt
2 tablespoons whole-wheat flour
½ teaspoon ground cumin
1 teaspoon salt
¼ cup nonfat milk
1 jalapeño, seeded and diced
4 Kim's Light Flat Bread™
¼ cup shredded low-fat Cheddar cheese
¾ cup shredded fat-free Cheddar cheese
Salsa, optional

Preheat the oven to 350° F. Combine the chicken, spinach, and scallions in a large bowl. Combine the sour cream, yogurt, flour, cumin, and salt in a medium bowl. Add the milk and jalapeño and mix well. Pour half of the sauce into the chicken mixture and mix well. Put 1 cup of filling on the center of each flat bread and roll up. Place the filled flat breads seam side down in a small, ungreased rectangular baking dish. Spoon the remaining sauce over the flat breads and bake for 20 minutes, or until heated through. Sprinkle with the cheeses and let stand for 5 minutes. Top with salsa and scallions, if desired, and serve.

Makes 8 servings; Serving size: ¹/₂ enchilada

PER SERVING: ■ ■ ■

Calories: 200	Total Carbs: 15 g
Total Fat: 3 g	Dietary Fiber: 4 g
Cholesterol: 50 mg	Protein: 30 g
Sodium: 771 mg	Sugar: 3 g

recipes

247

chickpea pot pie

I have to be honest, this is one I DIDN'T want to sample. Chickpea pot pie?! It tastes better, yes, better, than any warm comfort food casserole I've ever had, and no one has any idea that there are the dreaded (in the minds of my boys) chickpeas in it. OMGosh! It's now a favorite. Will I ever learn?

2 teaspoons grapeseed oil

1½ cups onion, diced

2 teaspoons cloves garlic, minced

1 cup celery, chopped

1 cup carrots, diced

3 cups low-sodium vegetable broth, divided

2 cups frozen corn kernels

One 15-ounce can garbanzo beans (chickpeas), rinsed and drained

2 tablespoons dried parsley

2 teaspoons each basil, marjoram, thyme

Salt and freshly ground black pepper

2 teaspoons cornstarch

1 tablespoon whole-wheat flour

2 ounces fat-free cream cheese

½ cup fat-free grated Parmesan cheese

1 cup frozen peas

1 cup frozen green beans

4 sheets frozen fillo, thawed

Fat-free spray butter

Heat oil in sauce pan over medium heat, add onion, and cook 15 minutes, until it browns. Stir in garlic, then celery and carrots and sauté 5 minutes. Stir in 2½ cups broth, corn, chickpeas, parsley, basil, marjoram, and thyme; season with salt and pepper to taste, if desired. Reduce heat to medium-low and simmer 30 minutes.

Whisk together cornstarch, flour, and remaining ½ cup broth. Stir cornstarch mixture, cream cheese, and Parmesan cheese into vegetable mixture. Season with salt and pepper, if desired. Remove from heat, and cool. Stir in peas and green beans.

Preheat oven to 370°F. Pour mixture into a pie plate. Crisscross each sheet of fillo squirting spray butter in between each layer and tucking in sides. Pierce top in several places with knife to allow steam to escape. Bake 30 to 40 minutes or until crust is flaky and brown.

Makes 12 servings; Serving size: ¹/₁₂ of pie

PER SERVING: ■■

Calories: 121	Total Carbs: 24 g
Total Fat: 1 g	Dietary Fiber: 5 g
Cholesterol: 1 mg	Protein: 6 g
Sodium: 571 mg	Sugar: 4 g

chicken cibolo

This is one of those recipes that takes you by surprise. I knew it was going to be good, but I had no idea how absolutely amazing it would turn out! Yummo!

24 ounces boneless skinless chicken breast halves

MARINADE:

1 large orange, peeled
2 tablespoons lime juice
One 8-ounce can pineapple
4 cloves garlic
2 tablespoons fresh rosemary
1 bay leaf

TOPPING:

6 ounces Cabot® reduced-fat Cheddar cheese
1½ cups of Mock Guac (see page 212)
3 ripe tomatoes, sliced into 24 slices (2 per sandwich)
4 cups finely shredded lettuce
One 21-ounce crusty French or Persian bread, sliced into
    1.75 ounces each or Persian bread, sliced into 1.75 ounces
    each
Butter-flavored cooking spray

Using a sharp knife, slice the chicken breast in a cross-section so that each piece is thin and weighs 2 ounces. If you are using the presliced, thin chicken breasts they may be less than 2 ounces each, so you will need to adjust accordingly.

In a food processor add, orange, lime juice, pineapple, and garlic and pulse until chopped. Add in rosemary and pulse a few more times. Pour into a zip-top bag and add chicken and bay leaf. Marinate in fridge for at least 1 hour (or overnight).

After marinating, grill over moderately hot coals until cooked through and no pink is left in chicken breast. Before removing from grill, place a slice of Cheddar cheese on each breast.

At this time spray bread slices lightly with butter-flavored cooking spray and toast the top side lightly. Flip the bread and place the chicken onto it. Top with 2 tomato slices and 2 tablespoons of the Mock Guac. Remove to a plate and sprinkle with ½ cup of finely shredded lettuce.

Makes 12 servings; Serving size: 1 chicken sandwich

PER SERVING: ■■■■■

Calories: 229	Total Carbs: 29 g
Total Fat: 5 g	Dietary Fiber: 1 g
Cholesterol: 41 mg	Protein: 23 g
Sodium: 480 mg	Sugar: 0 g

chicken divan

This great recipe was made at all of the Calvary Church get-togethers for years. Taste it and see why! Mmmmmmmm.

1½ pounds chicken breasts, cooked and cut into pieces
8 cups fresh broccoli florets, lightly steamed
Two 10¾-ounce cans 98-percent fat-free cream of
    mushroom soup
1 cup fat-free mayonnaise
3 teaspoons lemon juice
⅔ cup shredded reduced-fat Cheddar cheese
3½ ounces Kashi TLC Fire Roasted Veggie Crackers, crushed
2 tablespoons Brummel & Brown® Buttery Spread

Preheat the oven to 350°F. Place the chicken and broccoli on the bottom of a 9 × 13-inch baking dish. Mix the soup, mayonnaise, and lemon juice in a small bowl. Pour the sauce over the chicken and broccoli. Mix the cheese, cracker crumbs, and Brummel & Brown. Sprinkle over the casserole and bake for about 30 minutes, or until heated through.

Makes 16 servings; Serving size: ¹⁄₁₆ of recipe

PER SERVING: ■■

Calories: 130	Total Carbs: 13 g
Total Fat: 3 g	Dietary Fiber: 2 g
Cholesterol: 27 mg	Protein: 13 g
Sodium: 404 mg	Sugar: 1.5 g

cod with seafood stuffing

A very non-fishy-tasting dish that packs a ton of flavor.

Fat-free cooking spray
1 cup Pepperidge Farm Herb Stuffing Mix
⅓ cup plain bread crumbs
4 ounces crabmeat
7 ounces minced clams
¼ teaspoon garlic powder
¾ teaspoon dried parsley
¾ teaspoon dried basil
½ teaspoon dried oregano
Salt and freshly ground black pepper
Six 4-ounce cod fillets

Preheat the oven to 350° F. Spray a 9 × 13-inch baking dish with fat-free cooking spray. Prepare the stuffing mix, using the water drained from the crabmeat instead of tap water and omitting the butter. Mix the stuffing, bread crumbs, crabmeat, clams, garlic powder, parsley, basil, oregano, and salt and pepper to taste in a medium bowl. Lay the cod fillets in the dish. Spoon approximately ⅓ to ½ cup stuffing on top of each fillet. Wrap the ends of each fillet around the stuffing and secure with a toothpick. Bake uncovered for 20 minutes. Cover with foil and bake for another 10 minutes.

Makes 6 servings; Serving size: 1 stuffed fillet

PER SERVING: ■ ■ ■ ■ ■

Calories: 264	Total Carbs: 14 g
Total Fat: 5 g	Dietary Fiber: 2 g
Cholesterol: 100 mg	Protein: 38 g
Sodium: 482 mg	Sugar: 1 g

creamy baked chicken breasts

Chicken, stuffing, and gravy all in one! My husband's favorite.

Four 4-ounce chicken breasts, cut in half
4 ounces low-fat Swiss cheese, sliced
One 10¾-ounce can fat-free cream of chicken soup
¼ cup water
2 cups Stove Top stuffing mix, crushed
1 cup 98-percent fat-free chicken broth

Preheat the oven to 350° F. Arrange the chicken breasts side by side in a baking dish. Lay the Swiss cheese over the chicken. Combine the soup with ¼ cup water and pour over the chicken. Top with the stuffing mix and drizzle with the chicken broth. Bake uncovered for 45 to 50 minutes.

Makes 8 servings; Serving size: 2 ounces chicken and ¼ cup stuffing

PER SERVING: ■ ■ ■ ■

Calories: 208	Total Carbs: 12 g
Total Fat: 4 g	Dietary Fiber: 1 g
Cholesterol: 60 mg	Protein: 25 g
Sodium: 597 mg	Sugar: 2 g

LOW-CARB OPTION: Substitute 1 large slice lean ham for the stuffing mix and cut into 8 slices. Place some ham and Swiss cheese on each chicken breast and fold in half. Secure with a toothpick. Increase the cooking time by 5 minutes. Total carbs: 2.5 grams.

kim's light lasagna

The wraps make a great substitute for lasagna noodles without all the calories. I dare you to tell the difference. This recipe rocks!

1½ cups fat-free ricotta cheese
2 tablespoons chopped fresh parsley
2 ounces egg substitute
1 teaspoon dried oregano
1 teaspoon garlic salt
½ teaspoon garlic powder
½ teaspoon freshly ground black pepper
3¾ cups Meat Sauce (see page 256)
3 Kim's Light Flat Bread™
2 cups shredded fat-free mozzarella cheese
2 tablespoons grated fat-free Parmesan cheese

Preheat the oven to 350° F. Mix the ricotta, parsley, egg substitute, oregano, garlic salt, garlic powder, and pepper in a medium bowl. Layer the following ingredients in a 9 × 13-inch baking dish: ¾ cup Meat Sauce on the bottom of the pan, 1 Kim's Light Flat Bread, ½ of the ricotta mixture, and ⅓ of the mozzarella cheese. Repeat the layer, using 1½ cups Meat Sauce for each of the remaining layers. Finish the last layer with the last flat bread, the rest of the sauce, and the rest of the mozzarella. Sprinkle with Parmesan. Bake for 30 minutes. Remove from the oven and let stand for a few minutes before serving.

Makes 12 servings; Serving size: ¹⁄₁₂ of recipe

PER SERVING: ■■

Calories: 123	Total Carbs: 16 g
Total Fat: 2 g	Dietary Fiber: 2 g
Cholesterol: 17 mg	Protein: 14 g
Sodium: 743 mg	Sugar: 1 g

recipes

meat sauce

A quick and easy sauce that has great versatility. So much sauce! So few calories! I love to pour it over steamed broccoli.

¾ pound lean ground turkey
4 garlic cloves
Three 16-ounce cans tomato sauce
1 teaspoon dried oregano
1 teaspoon dried parsley
1 teaspoon dried basil
1 teaspoon sea salt
½ teaspoon freshly ground black pepper
1 bay leaf, broken in half

Brown the turkey in a pan. When the turkey is completely cooked, drain by pouring it through a strainer and then letting it sit on a few paper towels for 5 minutes. Put the remaining ingredients in a saucepot. Add the cooked turkey and bring to a simmer. Reduce the heat to low and simmer for about 45 minutes, stirring occasionally. Remove the bay leaf. Use immediately or freeze in an airtight container.

Makes 12 servings; Serving size: ½ cup

PER SERVING: ■

Calories: 62	Total Carbs: 6 g
Total Fat: 2 g	Dietary Fiber: 2 g
Cholesterol: 20 mg	Protein: 7 g
Sodium: 234 mg	Sugar: 4 g

mmmmmmmmeatloaf

The Rice Krispies add a lighter breading to the meatloaf and don't weigh it down—and this meatloaf doesn't weigh you down either.

½ pound lean ground beef
¾ pound lean ground turkey
4 ounces egg substitute
1¼ cups Kellogg's Rice Krispies cereal
1 teaspoon garlic salt
1 large onion, minced
¼ cup ketchup

Preheat the oven to 350° F. Mix all of the ingredients except the ketchup in a large bowl. Spread the mixture into a loaf pan and drizzle the ketchup on top. Bake for 60 to 75 minutes, or until the meat in the center is no longer pink.

Makes 8 servings; Serving size: 3 ounces

PER SERVING: ■ ■ ■ ■

Calories: 175	Total Carbs: 8 g
Total Fat: 9 g	Dietary Fiber: 1 g
Cholesterol: 51 mg	Protein: 16 g
Sodium: 215 mg	Sugar: 3 g

polynesian chicken

Thanks, Mom B., for this quick and delicious casserole.

    2 pounds boneless skinless chicken breasts
    ½ cup fat-free red Catalina or French dressing
    ½ cup sugar-free apricot preserves
    1 small envelope onion soup mix

Preheat the oven to 350° F. Wash the chicken, cut it into
2-inch pieces, and place the pieces in a 9 x 13-inch baking
dish. Mix the remaining ingredients and pour half of the sauce
over the chicken. Cover and bake for 45 minutes. Stir in the
remaining sauce and bake uncovered another 20 minutes.
Tender and savory!

Makes 8 servings; Serving size: ⅛ of recipe

PER SERVING: ■ ■ ■

Calories: 151	Total Carbs: 15 g
Total Fat: 1 g	Dietary Fiber: 0 g
Cholesterol: 65 mg	Protein: 23 g
Sodium: 606 mg	Sugar: 8 g

seafood newburg

This is a lightened version of my mom's original Maine Newburg. The original recipe called for so much butter, you could see pools of gold glistening on top of each bowl. Be still my beating heart . . . not anymore! And, in case you're interested, my mom loves this, too!

    12 ounces cooked shrimp (tails removed)
    12 ounces cooked lobster meat
    12 ounces raw scallops
    One can 98-percent fat-free condensed cream of celery soup
    ½ cup fat-free half & half
    7 ounces fat-free Cheddar cheese
    8 ounces white wine
    1 teaspoon parsley
    1 tablespoon cornstarch (mixed with ¼ cup cold water until
        dissolved)
    1 teaspoon desired seasoning (chipotle)

In a sauce pan add all the ingredients except the seafood. Bring to a boil, stirring constantly. Simmer on medium heat to reduce for 10 minutes. In a 9 x 13-inch baking dish, lay all the fish out and pour the sauce on top. Stir gently and cook at 350° F for 30 to 40 minutes until scallops are cooked and the sauce is thickened. Serve over veggies, rice, pasta, or enjoy as a bisque.

Makes 11 servings; Serving size: ¾ cup

PER SERVING: ■■■

Calories: 155	Total Carbs: 5 g
Total Fat: 1 g	Dietary Fiber: 0 g
Cholesterol: 97 mg	Protein: 25 g
Sodium: 536 mg	Sugar: 1 g

sesame chicken and slaw

This filling salad is really a hearty meal. Enjoy!

SLAW:

6 cups cabbage, sliced thin

1½ cups green bell peppers, sliced thin

1½ cups yellow or red bell peppers, sliced thin

1 cup snow peas, sliced thin

¼ cup scallions, chopped

1½ cups cucumber, peeled and spears

DRESSING:

½ cup white cooking wine

¼ cup white vinegar

¼ cup lite soy sauce

2 tablespoons ginger root, shredded

1 tablespoon low-calorie brown sugar*

2 teaspoons grapeseed oil

CHICKEN:

¼ cup Egg Beaters®

1 package Kikkoman® stir fry packet mixed with 2 tablespoons water

8 ounces chicken breast, no skin

¼ cup sesame seeds

SLAW: Toss together cabbage, bell peppers, snow peas, scallion, and cucumber in a large serving bowl for ginger slaw. Set aside.

DRESSING: In a separate bowl whisk together wine, vinegar, soy sauce, ginger, brown sugar, and grapeseed oil until brown sugar is dissolved. Set aside.

CHICKEN: Whisk together Egg Beaters and Kikkoman packet in a shallow bowl. Add chicken and turn until coated on all sides. Thread chicken onto skewers and sprinkle on the sesame seeds, coating well on all sides. Preheat oven to 350° F. Spray a cookie sheet with cooking spray, place skewers on the sheet and bake, turning occasionally, until browned on all sides and chicken is cooked through, about 15 minutes.

Pour dressing over ginger slaw and toss until well-coated. Serve with the warm chicken skewers.

Makes 8 servings; Serving size: 1 ounce chicken, 1½ cups of slaw

PER SERVING: ■■

Calories: 138	Total Carbs: 11 g
Total Fat: 4 g	Dietary Fiber: 3 g
Cholesterol: 16 mg	Protein: 11 g
Sodium: 608 mg	Sugar: 4 g

shredded pork

I had this recently at Uncle Arn and Aunt Helen's golden wedding anniversary and cousin Tom was sweet enough to share his recipe. It's light and fabulously tasty and all, but melts in your mouth.

22 ounces pork tenderloin, cut into chunks
1 cup chopped onion
1 green bell pepper, minced
1½ teaspoons dried oregano
2 teaspoons garlic salt
¼ teaspoon freshly ground black pepper
¼ teaspoon garlic powder
2 teaspoons minced garlic
½ cup water

Put all the ingredients together in a slow cooker and set on high for 20 minutes. Then change to the low setting and leave for 14 hours. Check every 2 hours and as you stir it around, start pulling the meat apart with forks. As it cooks slowly it will begin to fall apart. In the end you will have fabulous shredded pork. Serve with a side of barbecue sauce and low-calorie rolls to make pork sandwiches.

Makes 6 servings; Serving size: about ¾ cup

PER SERVING: ■ ■ ■ ■

Calories: 196	Total Carbs: 4 g
Total Fat: 6 g	Dietary Fiber: 1 g
Cholesterol: 82 mg	Protein: 29 g
Sodium: 834 mg	Sugar: 0 g

spinach-stuffed chicken breasts

I just love anything stuffed . . . except me!

   Fat-free cooking spray
   4 slices Oscar Mayer® precooked bacon, diced
   4 garlic cloves, minced
   1 cup finely chopped onions
   One 10-ounce package frozen chopped spinach, thawed
      and well drained
   ¼ cup egg substitute
   1 ounce fat-free garlic and onion croutons, crushed
   2 teaspoons dried rosemary, crushed
   1 ounce roasted red bell pepper, packed in water, drained
      and chopped
   Eight 4-ounce skinless chicken breasts
   Salt and freshly ground black pepper
   2 teaspoons Brummel & Brown® Buttery Spread®
   Lemon wedges

In a nonstick frying pan sprayed lightly with fat-free cooking
spray, sauté the bacon, garlic, and onions lightly for about
2 minutes. Transfer to a large bowl. Add the spinach, egg
substitute, croutons, rosemary, and bell pepper and mix well.
With a sharp knife, cut a pocket in the thick side of each
chicken breast. Stuff lightly with the spinach mixture and
close with a wooden toothpick if needed. Season the stuffed
chicken breasts lightly with salt and pepper. In the same pan
over medium heat, melt the Brummel & Brown. Add the
chicken breasts and cook for 20 to 25 minutes, turning occasionally until done. Remove the toothpicks and serve with
lemon wedges.

Makes 8 servings; Serving size: 1 stuffed chicken breast

PER SERVING: ■ ■ ■ ■

Calories: 191	Total Carbs: 9 g
Total Fat: 3 g	Dietary Fiber: 2 g
Cholesterol: 72 mg	Protein: 30 g
Sodium: 563 mg	Sugar: 1 g

recipes

thai beef skewers

Great for an appetizer or a main meal!

MARINADE:

½ cup soy sauce

½ teaspoon ground ginger

1 teaspoon canola oil

2 teaspoons crushed garlic

½ teaspoon lime juice

2 tablespoons brown sugar substitute

¼ cup water

18 ounces very lean round steak, sliced into ⅛-inch-thick strips

Mix all of the ingredients, except the steak, with ¼ cup water in a small bowl. Thread the steak strips onto wooden skewers. Feel free to add whatever veggies you'd like, not factored. Lay the prepared skewers in a shallow dish. Drizzle half of the marinade on top and let stand for about 30 minutes. Reserve the remaining liquid for dipping sauce. Lay the skewers on a broiler pan and broil for several minutes on each side, or until the steak is done to your preference. These can be cooked on a grill as well. Serve with the reserved sauce.

Makes 6 servings; Serving size: 3-ounce skewer

PER SERVING: ■ ■ ■

Calories: 153	Total Carbs: 6 g
Total Fat: 4 g	Dietary Fiber: 0 g
Cholesterol: 49 mg	Protein: 21 g
Sodium: 1,243 mg	Sugar: 4 g

whole-wheat pizza dough

I think I've died and gone to heaven. Finally, a pizza crust that fits my diet. Use it as a pizza crust. Use it as a calzone. Be creative. This is a great dough and makes two recipes!

1 cup lukewarm water
2 teaspoons sugar substitute
1 package active dry yeast
3 cups whole-wheat flour
1 teaspoon salt
5 teaspoons olive oil
Fat-free cooking spray

Combine 1 cup lukewarm water, sugar substitute, and yeast in a small bowl. Let stand until foamy (about 5 minutes). Sift together 2½ cups of the flour and the salt. Slowly add the yeast mixture and the oil while mixing on low speed for 3 minutes. The dough should be thoroughly blended in a slightly sticky ball. Turn onto a lightly floured surface and knead for 5 to 6 minutes, adding the remaining ½ cup flour to prevent sticking, until smooth and elastic. Shape into a ball. Place in a glass bowl sprayed with fat-free cooking spray and cover with plastic wrap. Let rise in a warm place until doubled in size, about 1 hour. Punch down the dough and shape into two balls. The dough can be stored in a zip-top bag with the excess air pressed out, refrigerated overnight, or frozen for up to a month. The dough must be at room temperature before shaping.

Preheat the oven to 350° F. Add sauce, veggies, cheese, and other toppings (not included in nutritional info). Bake for 30 minutes.

Makes 2 pizza crusts; Serving size: 1 slice, 8 slices each pizza crust

PER SERVING: ■

Calories: 90	Total Carbs: 17 g
Total Fat: 2 g	Dietary Fiber: 3 g
Cholesterol: 0 mg	Protein: 3 g
Sodium: 146 mg	Sugar: 0 g

desserts

2-minute mug cake

Portion control is key to any success to weight loss, but so is knowing which are your trigger foods. Cake happens to be mine. This 2-Minute Mug Cake hits the spot and I don't have to deal with leftovers . . . or mixing bowls.

3½ tablespoons cake flour
4 tablespoons canned pumpkin
1 tablespoon powdered cocoa
1 tablespoon Egg Beaters®
3 tablespoons Splenda®
¼ teaspoon baking soda
¼ teaspoon baking powder
½ teaspoon vanilla

Mix all ingredients in a microwave-safe mug. Cook it for 2 minutes on high. Carefully remove and enjoy!

Makes 1 serving; Serving size: 1 cake

PER SERVING: ■■
_____

Calories: 135
Total Fat: 1 g
Cholesterol: 0 mg
Sodium: 470 mg

Total Carbs: 28 g
Dietary Fiber: 4 g
Protein: 6 g
Sugar: 3 g
_____

apple cake

This cake is so moist . . . and makes your kitchen smell delish!

Fat-free cooking spray
1½ cups sugar substitute
6 cups apples, peeled, cored, and cubed
4 ounces egg substitute
1 cup unsweetened applesauce
3 cups all-purpose flour
1 teaspoon salt
1½ teaspoons ground cinnamon
2 teaspoons baking soda
1 teaspoon grated nutmeg
⅓ cup raisins

Preheat the oven to 350° F. Spray a bundt pan or a 9 × 13-inch pan with fat-free cooking spray. Pour the sugar substitute over the apples and let stand for 10 minutes. Add the egg substitute and applesauce and mix well. Mix in the flour, salt, cinnamon, baking soda, nutmeg, and raisins. Pour the batter into the prepared pan. Bake for 50 minutes.

Makes 18 servings; Serving size: ¹⁄₁₈ of cake

PER SERVING: ■■

Calories: 120	Total Carbs: 29 g
Total Fat: 0 g	Dietary Fiber: 2 g
Cholesterol: 0 mg	Protein: 3 g
Sodium: 283 mg	Sugar: 2 g

recipes

apple crumb

Crumbled fillo dough gives this topping the crunch that satisfies. Great for the fall or any time of the year.

    5 apples, peeled and chopped
    2 tablespoons sugar substitute, divided
    2 tablespoons brown sugar substitute
    1 tablespoon plus 1 teaspoon pumpkin pie spice
    2 teaspoons lemon juice
    4 ounces fillo dough, dried and crumbled
    Fat-free spray butter

Preheat the oven to 425°F. Combine the apples, 1 tablespoon sugar substitute, brown sugar substitute, 1 tablespoon pumpkin pie spice, and lemon juice in a large bowl. Mix well. Fill a 9-inch pie plate or a 9-inch square baking dish.

In a frying pan, mix the fillo, 1 teaspoon pumpkin pie spice, and 1 tablespoon sugar substitute. Cook over medium heat for 5 to 7 minutes. Spray the fillo with 40 pumps of fat-free spray butter and mix well. Just as it is crumbling more, remove from the heat and cover the apples evenly. Bake for 6 minutes. Decrease the oven temperature to 350°F and bake for 35 minutes.

Makes 8 servings; Serving size: ⅛ of dish

PER SERVING: ■■

Calories: 112	Total Carbs: 25 g
Total Fat: 1 g	Dietary Fiber: 3 g
Cholesterol: 0 mg	Protein: 1 g
Sodium: 69 mg	Sugar: 3 g

cobb family marble cheesecake

This recipe goes back to the early 1900s in Portland, Maine. My great-grandmother made them and my great-grandfather rowed from ship to ship selling them along with other grocery items to the moored ships' captains. Make this fat free or substitute low-fat dairy products for a firmer cheesecake, but make sure you make it!

CRUST:

¼ cup Fiber One cereal
½ cup Cocoa Puffs cereal
Fat-free cooking spray

FILLING:

½ cup reduced-fat cream cheese
½ cup fat-free cream cheese
2 teaspoons vanilla extract
4 ounces egg substitute
1½ cups fat-free sour cream
1 tablespoon all-purpose flour
2 tablespoons unsweetened cocoa powder
½ cup sugar substitute
¼ cup chocolate syrup

Preheat the oven to 350°F.

CRUST: Put the cereals in the bowl of a food processor and process until fine. Spray the bottom of a 6-inch springform pan lightly with fat-free cooking spray. Sprinkle the crust evenly across the bottom of the pan. (No butter is needed.)

FILLING: Mix the cream cheeses in a food processor. Add the vanilla, egg substitute, sour cream, flour, cocoa powder, and sugar substitute and mix until well blended. Pour evenly on top of the crust. Drizzle the chocolate syrup on top and pull a knife through to swirl the chocolate; don't push the knife in too deep, to avoid moving the crust. Bake for about 1¼ hours, or until the top is firm to the touch and just starts to brown.

The top may crack slightly. Refrigerate for at least 4 hours. I wrap it in a clean linen dish towel in the refrigerator, which keeps moisture from forming on the top. Run a knife around the edges before releasing the cake from the pan. This can be served on the springform base.

Makes 8 servings; Serving size: $\frac{1}{8}$ of cake

PER SERVING: ■■
___

Calories: 108

Total Fat: 3 g

Cholesterol: 10 mg

Sodium: 214 mg

Total Carbs: 14 g

Dietary Fiber: 3 g

Protein: 7 g

Sugar: 7 g
___

Suggested topping: fat-free whipped topping sprinkled lightly with cocoa powder.

crustless pumpkin pie

Go ahead, have seconds . . . or thirds!

    Fat-free cooking spray
    One 15-ounce can pumpkin
    ¾ cup sugar substitute
    ½ cup egg substitute
    1½ cups skim milk
    ½ teaspoon salt
    2 tablespoons pumpkin pie spice
    1 tablespoon flour

Preheat the oven to 400° F. Spray a 9-inch glass or microwave-safe pie plate lightly with fat-free cooking spray. Beat all of the ingredients together. Pour the batter into the pie plate and bake for 15 minutes. Decrease the oven temperature to 350° F and bake for another 45 minutes. Cook on high in microwave for additional 2 minutes, or until knife inserted in the center comes out clean. Top with a dollop of fat-free whipped cream (not factored).

Makes 4 servings; Serving size: ¼ of pie

PER SERVING: ■

Calories: 64	Total Carbs: 17 g
Total Fat: 0 g	Dietary Fiber: 1 g
Cholesterol: 2 mg	Protein: 4 g
Sodium: 893 mg	Sugar: 1 g

fat-free pound cake

I love that we found a way to make fat-free pound cake. Now you really can have your cake and EAT it, too!

  4 egg whites, whipped
  1 cup fat-free sour cream
  1 teaspoon vanilla
  1½ cups unbleached flour
  ½ cup granulated sugar
  ½ cup Splenda®
  ¼ teaspoon baking powder
  ¼ teaspoon baking soda

Preheat the oven at 325°F. Prepare a 9x5x3-inch pan with cooking spray and dust with flour. In a large bowl, whip egg whites until frothy and peaks begin to form. Combine sour cream and vanilla, and continue mixing. In another bowl, combine flour, sugar, Splenda, baking powder, and baking soda. Mix dry ingredients with wet ingredients just until moistened. Spread batter into prepared pan. Bake for 1 hour or until cake tests done.

Makes 12 servings; Serving size: 1/12 of loaf

PER SERVING: ■■

Calories: 128	Total Carbs: 29 g
Total Fat: 0 g	Dietary Fiber: 0 g
Cholesterol: 0 mg	Protein: 3 g
Sodium: 115 mg	Sugar: 17 g

fruit pizza

I gained about 80 of my 212 pounds eating the original version of this family recipe, which includes white chocolate chips and heavy cream. When I serve this lightened version to my family, they are just as thrilled as ever. A July Fourth favorite!

CRUST:

Fat-free butter-flavored cooking spray
10 large sheets fillo dough

GLAZE:

1 tablespoon cornstarch
¼ cup sugar substitute
½ teaspoon lemon juice
½ cup pineapple juice

FILLING:

8 ounces fat-free cream cheese
½ teaspoon lemon juice
2 tablespoons sugar-free, fat-free instant white chocolate
   pudding mix
½ cup sugar substitute
3 tablespoons nonfat milk
2 cups assorted berries and banana slices

Preheat the oven to 350° F.

CRUST: Spray a 12-inch pizza pan lightly with butter-flavored cooking spray. Lay 1 fillo sheet on half of the pan and spray it lightly with cooking spray. Lay another sheet on the other half, overlapping the sheets in the center. Continue spraying lightly and laying all of the fillo sheets around the pizza pan. Turn under any fillo dough hanging over the edges of the dish. Bake for 8 to 10 minutes, or until golden brown. Cool completely.

GLAZE: Mix the cornstarch, sugar substitute, ½ teaspoon lemon juice, and pineapple juice in a small saucepan. When thoroughly blended, heat over medium heat until the mixture thickens, stirring constantly. Cool.

FILLING: In a medium bowl beat the cream cheese, ½ teaspoon lemon juice, pudding mix, sugar substitute, and milk until smooth. Spread the cream cheese mixture on the crust very carefully, almost to the edge of the dough. Arrange the assorted fruit on top of the filling. Brush the glaze over the top of the fruit, making sure all the banana slices are covered to keep them from browning. Chill until ready to serve. Use a pizza slicer to cut the pizza into 8 large slices.

Makes 8 servings; Serving size: ⅛ of pizza

PER SERVING: ■■

Calories: 113	Total Carbs: 24 g
Total Fat: 0 g	Dietary Fiber: 1 g
Cholesterol: 5 mg	Protein: 7 g
Sodium: 305 mg	Sugar: 4 g

haystacks

Give that chocolate urge some satisfaction. If you're a chocoholic like my sister, Heather, whip up a batch of haystacks!

5½ ounces semisweet chocolate chips
1 teaspoon peanut butter
1½ cups Fiber One cereal
1 teaspoon sugar substitute

Heat the chocolate chips and peanut butter in a microwavable bowl until melted. Add the cereal and mix until completely coated. Drop by teaspoons onto wax paper and sprinkle with a little sugar substitute. Refrigerate until firm. You can make 8 large haystacks or 16 smaller ones.

Makes 8 servings; Serving size: 2 small haystacks

PER SERVING: ■

Calories: 80	Total Carbs: 14 g
Total Fat: 4 g	Dietary Fiber: 4 g
Cholesterol: 0 mg	Protein: 1 g
Sodium: 36 mg	Sugar: 7 g

key lime pie

⅓ cup boiling water
One 44-ounce box sugar-free lime gelatin
Two 6-ounce containers fat-free Key lime yogurt
8 ounces fat-free whipped topping
Kim's Light Pie Crust (see below)

Dissolve gelatin thoroughly in boiling water. Fold in yogurt and whipped topping. Pour filling into pie crust and chill at least 3 hours before serving.

Makes 8 servings; Serving size: ⅛ pie

PER SERVING: ■■

Calories: 109	Total Carbs: 30 g
Total Fat: 1 g	Dietary Fiber: 1 g
Cholesterol: 0 mg	Protein: 2 g
Sodium: 109 mg	Sugar: 18 g

Change up the flavors . . . strawberry, blueberry, lemon. Make your family's favorite flavor.

kim's light pie crust

Love those premade light graham cracker crusts. Hate their calories (yeah, even the light ones). Here's the solution.

1½ tablespoon Brummel & Brown® Buttery Spread, melted
1½ Kim's Light Bagels®, toasted and finely ground
½ cup brown sugar substitute
1 teaspoon cinnamon (optional, not factored)

To make crumbs, mix melted Brummel & Brown with ground light bagels and brown sugar substitute, until well-blended. Use hands to break apart the chunks. Spray a 9-inch pie plate with fat-free butter-flavored cooking spray. Evenly spread the crumbs on the bottom and sides of the pie plate. Use the back of a spoon or your fingers to press the crumbs into the pie plate. Bake at 400° F for 15 minutes. Remove from heat and allow to cool completely.

Makes 8 servings; Serving size: 1/8 of pie crust

PER SERVING: ■

Calories: 37	Total Carbs: 16 g
Total Fat: 1 g	Dietary Fiber: 1 g
Cholesterol: 0 mg	Protein: 0 g
Sodium: 47 mg	Sugar: 12 g

Note: You can use Kim's Light Bagels in Plain, Cinnamon, or Blueberry for this recipe.

midnight brownies

Dr. Oz liked this so much, he asked me to come on his show and make a version of it for him. He had no idea what the secret ingredient was that makes this brownie so moist and full of fiber. Your critics won't either!

BROWNIE:

One 15-ounce can black beans, drained and rinsed
¾ cup Splenda®
½ cup self-rising flour
¾ cup Egg Beaters®
¼ cup unsweetened cocoa
1 teaspoon vanilla
1 teaspoon baking powder
6 tablespoons semisweet mini chocolate chips

FROSTING:

3 ounces fat-free cream cheese
3 ounces reduced fat cream cheese
1 cup Splenda®
1 teaspoon vanilla

GLAZE:

2 tablespoons semisweet mini chocolate chips, melted.

Preheat the oven to 350° F. Lightly spray an 8 x 8-inch baking dish with nonstick cooking spray.

BROWNIE: In a food processor or blender, mix all brownie ingredients (except chocolate chips) together. Puree on high, for 1½ minutes or more, but it should be smooth. Clean off sides and blend for another 20 seconds. Fold in 6 tablespoons of chocolate chips. Spread into prepared dish. Bake for 20 minutes, until toothpick comes out clean. Cool.

FROSTING: Beat all ingredients until light and fluffy. Spread evenly over the top of the cooled brownies.

GLAZE: In a microwave-safe bowl, melt 2 tablespoons of chocolate chips with a 2-second spray of nonstick cooking oil. Using a spoon, swirl the chocolate on top of the frosted brownies. Allow it to set in the refrigerator for 20 minutes.

Makes 12 servings; Serving size: $\frac{1}{12}$ of recipe

PER SERVING: ■■

Calories: 129	Total Carbs: 17 g
Total Fat: 4 g	Dietary Fiber: 3 g
Cholesterol: 5 mg	Protein: 6 g
Sodium: 217 mg	Sugar: 6 g

peach cheesecake ice cream

This has such a refreshing, light flavor that everyone will love. Easy to make ice cream—without a machine—it doesn't get much better than that!

> 1 cup fat-free half & half
> Two 6-ounce containers DANNON® Light & Fit® Vanilla Yogurt
> 1 cup Low-Calorie Granulated Sugar*
> One 8-ounce package fat-free cream cheese
> 1 cup peaches, peeled and mashed

Using an electric mixer, blend first four ingredients until smooth. Stir in peaches. Place the bowl in an ice-water bath. Once the mixture has cooled, cover with plastic wrap and allow the mixture to age in the refrigerator for at least 4 hours or up to 24 hours. This aging process will give the mixture better whipping qualities and produce ice cream with more body and a smoother texture. After aging (chilling) the mixture, remove from the refrigerator and stir the mixture. The ice cream is now ready for the freezing process.

Transfer the ice cream mixture to a freezer-safe bowl or container if not already in an appropriate one. Cover tightly with plastic wrap, foil, or an airtight cover. Place the container in the freezer and allow the mixture to freeze for 2 hours. Remove from the freezer and beat with a hand mixer to break up ice crystals that are beginning to form. Cover and place back in the freezer. Freeze for 2 more hours and then remove from the freezer and beat again with the hand mixer. The ice cream should be thick but too soft to scoop. If it is not thick enough, return it to the freezer for additional freezing time. Pour into a plastic airtight freezer container. Pack the ice cream in the container. Be sure to leave at least ½ inch head space for expansion. Cover and place the container in the freezer and allow the ice cream to freeze until firm.

After the ice cream has hardened sufficiently, take the ice cream container out of the freezer, remove the cover and scoop ice cream into bowls or cones. Serve and enjoy!

Makes 8 servings; Serving size: ½ cup

PER SERVING: ■■

Calories: 103	Total Carbs: 35 g
Total Fat: 0 g	Dietary Fiber: 1 g
Cholesterol: 5 mg	Protein: 6 g
Sodium: 234 mg	Sugar: 30 g

penny's rich chocolate cake

Mmmm, mmmm, mmmmm! You go, girl!

Fat-free cooking spray
One 18¼-ounce box chocolate cake mix
One 1-ounce package sugar-free, fat-free chocolate
   pudding mix
16 ounces fat-free sour cream
½ cup nonfat milk
¼ cup water

Preheat the oven to 350° F. Lightly spray a nonstick Bundt pan with fat-free cooking spray. With an electric mixer, mix all of the ingredients until smooth. Spread the batter into the pan. Bake for 40 minutes. The tester will not come out clean, but make sure the cake is set.

Makes 18 servings; Serving size: ¹⁄₁₈ of cake

PER SERVING: ■■
_____

Calories: 125
Total Fat: 2 g
Cholesterol: 4 mg
Sodium: 255 mg

Total Carbs: 24 g
Dietary Fiber: 1 g
Protein: 2 g
Sugar: 13 g
_____

pumpkin pinwheels

This recipe only looks difficult. It's really so easy!

Fat-free cooking spray
One 16-ounce box angel food cake mix
One 15-ounce can pumpkin
1 tablespoon pumpkin pie spice
8 ounces fat-free cream cheese
¼ cup sugar substitute, plus more for sprinkling the towel
2 teaspoons vanilla extract

Preheat the oven to 350° F. Lightly spray a rimmed nonstick baking sheet with fat-free cooking spray. Combine the cake mix, pumpkin, and pumpkin pie spice in a bowl. You will notice the chemical reaction almost immediately. Spread the batter on the baking sheet. Bake for 20 minutes, or until the cake springs back lightly to the touch. Lay a damp linen towel on the counter, sprinkled lightly with sugar substitute. Go around the edges of the cake with a spatula to make sure it isn't sticking to the pan. Turn the slightly cooked cake onto the prepared towel. Roll up the towel, the long way, with the cake inside. Place the cake in the refrigerator and let cool. Meanwhile, blend the cream cheese, sugar substitute, and vanilla with an electric mixer. When the cake has cooled, unroll it and spread with the cream cheese mixture. Immediately roll the cake back up (without the towel). Wrap in plastic wrap and refrigerate until ready to serve. Cut the roll from the center out, making equal parts.

Makes 16 servings; Serving size: ¹⁄₁₆ of the recipe

PER SERVING: ■■

Calories: 130	Total Carbs: 27 g
Total Fat: 0 g	Dietary Fiber: 1 g
Cholesterol: 2 mg	Protein: 5 g
Sodium: 327 mg	Sugar: 19 g

tiramisu

A light or low-fat pound cake can be used instead. But be sure to add in the additional calories—nothing's lighter than ours (see page 272)!

½ cup Splenda®, divided
2 teaspoons vanilla extract
8 ounces mascarpone cheese
½ cup fat-free ricotta cheese
¼ cup low-fat whipped cream cheese
2 tablespoons cocoa powder
6 tablespoons hot water
2 teaspoons instant espresso or coffee
1 fat-free pound cake (see page 272)

In a medium bowl mix ¼ cup of Splenda®, vanilla, and mascarpone cheese. On slow speed, add ricotta cheese and cream cheese, until well-blended and spreadable. In a small bowl combine remaining ¼ cup of Splenda®, water, and instant coffee. Stir until all dissolved. Cut the pound cake down to be 8 inches in length. Lay on its side, trim off the rounded top (not too much) and make 4 equal strips. Lay on the bottom of an 8 x 8-inch baking dish. Using the "scraps" fill in any holes. Top with ½ of the espresso mixture and ½ of the cheese mixture. Sprinkle ⅓ of the cocoa powder. Repeat steps of cake, the espresso mixture, the cheese mixture, and ⅓ of the cocoa powder. Chill for 1 hour. Just before serving sprinkle the rest of the cocoa. Discard any leftover cake or use it to fill in any gaps.

Makes 12 servings; Serving size: ¹⁄₁₂ of loaf

PER SERVING: ■ ■ ■ ■

Calories: 157	Total Carbs: 18 g
Total Fat: 8 g	Dietary Fiber: 1 g
Cholesterol: 22 mg	Protein: 3 g
Sodium: 133 mg	Sugar: 7 g

BAKERY/DELI/PRODUCE

- Alouette Cucumber Dill Spread
  cal 50 | fat 4g | fib 0g | carb 2g • serving size 2 tbsp | ■

- Alouette Lite Garlic & Herb Spread
  cal 50 | fat 3.5g | fib 0g | carb 2g • serving size 2 tbsp | ■

- Et Tu Salad Kit—Light Caesar
  cal 80 | fat 6g | fib 0g | carb 6g • serving size 1/6 container | ■ ■

- Hill & Valley Angel Food Cake, Sugar Free
  cal 60 | fat 0g | fib 2g | carb 19g • serving size 1/6 | ■

* • Isabella's Angel Food Cake, Sugar Free
  cal 90 | fat 0g | fib 5g | carb 26g • serving size 1/5 cake | ■

* • Marzetto Fat Free Ranch & Dill Veggie Dips
  cal 30 | fat 5g | fib 0g | carb 3g • serving size 2 tbsp | ■

* • Mira Light Mango Nectar
  cal 65 | fat 0g | fib 1g | carb 17g • serving size 8 oz | ■

- Sensible Choice Angel Food Cake, Sugar Free
  cal 90 | fat 0g | fib 5g | carb 29g • serving size 1/5 cake | ■

* • Wholly Guacamole 100 Calorie Snack Packs
  cal 100 | fat 8g | fib 4g | carb 5g • serving size 1 packet | ■ ■

SNACKS/POPCORN/CHIPS

- Athenos Baked Whole Wheat Pita Chips
  cal 120 | fat 4g | fib 2g | carb 18g • serving size 11 chips | ■ ■

- Blue Ginger Multi-Grain Brown Rice Chips
  cal 110 | fat 3g | fib 3g | carb 21g • serving size 33 chips | ■ ■

- Curves Strawberries & Cream Granola Bar
  cal 100 | fat 2g | fib 5g | carb 19g • serving size 1 bar | ■

- Emerald Coco Roast Almonds 100 cal packs
  cal 100 | fat 8g | fib 2g | carb 4g • serving size 1 pack | ■ ■

*Kim's favorites!

- Guiltless Gourmet Tortilla Chips
  cal 120 | fat 2g | fib 2g | carb 19g • serving size 1 oz | ■ ■

* • Healthy Pop Jolly Time 94% FF Micro Popcorn
  cal 90 | fat 2g | fib 9g | carb 23g • serving size 1/2 large bag | ■

- Kavli Garlic Crispbreads
  cal 83 | fat 2g | fib 3g | carb 17g •· serving size 5 pieces | ■

- Kernel Season's Popcorn Seasonings
  cal 2 | fat 0g | fib 0g | carb 0g • serving size 1/4 tsp | □

* • Lays Light Potato Chips (plain & barbecue)
  cal 75 | fat 0g | fib 1g | carb 17g • serving size 1 oz | ■

* • Natures Place Soy Chips
  cal 120 | fat 4g | fib 1g | carb 20g • serving size 1 oz/19 crisps | ■ ■

- NY Flat Bread
  cal 50 | fat 1.5g | fib <0g | carb 7g • serving size 1 piece | ■

- NY Style Mini 96% Fat Free Garlic Bagel Chips
  cal 70 | fat 1g | fib 1g | carb 14g • serving size 22 pieces | ■

- Old London Melba Snacks
  cal 50 | fat 1g | fib 1g | carb 11g • serving size 4 pieces | ■

- Orville Redenbacher's Smart Pop 94% Fat Free
  cal 120 | fat 2g | fib 4g | carb 25g • serving size 1/2 large bag | ■ ■

* • Pringles Baked Wheat Stix (assorted flavors)
  cal 90 | fat 4g | fib 0g | carb 11g • serving size 1 pack | ■ ■

- Pringles Light Fat Free
  cal 70 | fat 0g | fib 1g | carb 15g • serving size 15 pieces | ■

- Quaker Quakes (assorted flavors)
  cal 60 | fat 1g | fib 0g | carb 13g • serving size 7 mini cakes | ■

* • Ruffles Light Potato Chips (plain & cheddar/sour cream)
  cal 75 | fat 0g | fib 1g | carb 17g • serving size 1 oz | ■

- Smartfood Reduced Fat White Cheddar Popcorn
  cal 47 | fat 2g | fib 1g | carb 6g • serving size 1 cup | ■

- Snack Factory Pretzel Crisps (assorted flavors)
  cal 110 | fat 0g | fib 1g | carb 23g • serving size 11 crisps | ■ ■

- Soytato Chips
  cal 120 | fat 3g | fib 2g | carb 16g • serving size 26 chips | ■ ■

* • Special K Crackers
  cal 120 | fat 2g | fib 3g | carb 23g • serving size 30 crackers | ■ ■

- Tostitos Scoops, Baked
  cal 120 | fat 3g | fib 2g | carb 22g • serving size 1 oz (15 scoops) | ■■
- Trader Joe's VERY Mini Vanilla Meringues
  cal 100 | fat 0g | fib 0g | carb 24g • serving size 100 pieces | ■■
- Tree of Life Natural Wasabi Peas
  cal 120 | fat 4g | fib 2g | carb 17g • serving size 1/4 cup | ■■
- Triscuit Thin Crisps
  cal 130 | fat 5g | fib 3g | carb 21g • serving size 15 crackers | ■■
- Weight Watchers Frosted Snack Cakes (asst'd varieties)
  cal 80 | fat 2.5g | fib 2g | carb 16g • serving size 1 cake | ■

GROCERIES

- Alessi Rosemary Breadsticks
  cal 110 | fat 1.5g | fib 1g | carb 22g • serving size 9 sticks | ■■
- B&M No Sugar Added Homestyle Baked Beans
  cal 120 | fat 0g | fib 8g | carb 23g • serving size 1/2 cup | ■■
- Beef Jerky, Harley-Davidson
  cal 80 | fat 1g | fib 1g | carb 4g • serving size 1 oz | ■
- Betty Crocker Wild Blueberry Muffin Mix
  cal 128 | fat 1.8g | fib 0g | carb 26g • serving size 1 muffin | ■■
- Bidgford Turkey Pepperoni
  cal 80 | fat 4g | fib 0g | carb 1g • serving size 12 slices | ■■
- Bidgford Turkey Summer Sausage
  cal 90 | fat 5g | fib 0g | carb 1g • serving size 2 oz | ■■
- Biscotti Brothers Chocolate Almond Biscotti
  cal 100 | fat 3g | fib 1g | carb 15g • serving size 1 oz | ■■
- Bogdon's Chocolate Dipped Confections
  cal 53 | fat 1g | fib 0g | carb 10g • serving size 3 sticks | ■
- Bumble Bee Chicken Breast with seasonings
  cal 120 | fat 1g | fib 0g | carb 0g • serving size 4 oz foil pouch | ■■
- Bumble Bee Skinless/Boneless Pink Salmon
  cal 90 | fat 5g | fib 0g | carb 0g • serving size 2.2 oz drained | ■■
* - Campbell's Soup at Hand, Chicken & Stars
  cal 70 | fat 2g | fib 1g | carb 10g • serving size 1 container | ■
- Campbell's Soup at Hand, Classic Tomato
  cal 120 | fat 0g | fib 2g | carb 27g • serving size 1 container | ■■

- Campbell's Soup at Hand, Italian Style Wedding
  cal 90 | fat 4.5g | fib 2g | carb 10g • serving size 1 container | ■

- Campbell's Soup at Hand, Vegetable Beef
  cal 70 | fat 1g | fib 1g | carb 10g • serving size 1 container | ■

* • Campbell's 98% Fat Free Cream of Mushroom Soup
  cal 70 | fat 2.5g | fib 1g | carb 9g • serving size 1/2 cup | ■

* • Chatham Village Fat Free Garlic & Onion Croutons
  cal 60 | fat 0g | fib 0g | carb 10g • serving size 4 tbsp | ■

- Chi-Chi's Medium Salsa Snackers
  cal 35 | fat 0g | fib 1g | carb 8g • serving size 1 snacker cup | ■

- Del Monte—No Sugar Added Diced Fruit Cups
  cal 25–40 | fat 0g | fib 0g | carb 6–12g • serving size 1 snack cup | ■

- Fiber One Bran Cereal
  cal 60 | fat 1g | fib 14g | carb 25g • serving size 1/2 cup | □

- General Foods International Chai Latte
  cal 30 | fat 2g | fib 0g | carb 2g • serving size 1 tbsp | ■

- Gerber Graduate Mini Fruits
  cal 25 | fat 0g | fib 1g | carb 6g • serving size 1/4 cup | □

- Gerber Graduate Puffs
  cal 25 | fat 0g | fib 0g | carb 6g • serving size 73 pieces | □

- Healthy Choice Traditional Pasta Sauce
  cal 60 | fat 0g | fib 3g | carb 13g • serving size 1/2 cup | ■

- Healthy Request Chicken Rice Soup
  cal 70 | fat 1.5g | fib 1g | carb 13g • serving size 1/2 cup | ■

- Healthy Request Minestrone Soup
  cal 80 | fat .5g | fib 3g | carb 15g • serving size 1/2 cup | ■

- Heinz One Carb Ketchup
  cal 5 | fat 0g | fib 0g | carb 1g • serving size 1 tbsp | □

- Hershey's Lite Chocolate Syrup
  cal 45 | fat 0g | fib 0g | carb 11g • serving size 2 tbsp | ■

- Hershey's Sticks (milk chocolate, mint, or caramel filled)
  cal 60 | fat 3.5g | fib 0g | carb 6g • serving size 1 stick | ■

- Hodgson Mill Whole Wheat Gingerbread Mix
  cal 110 | fat 0g | fib 2g | carb 24g • serving size ¼ of the mix | ■ ■

- Hodgson Mill Whole Wheat Muffin Mix
  cal 130 | fat .5g | fib 3g | carb 27g • serving size 1 muffin | ■ ■

- Hormel Real Crumbled Bacon, 50% Reduced Fat
  cal 50 | fat 3g | fib 0g | carb 0g • serving size 2 tbsp | ■

* • Hostess 100 Calorie Chocolate Cupcakes
  cal 100 | fat 3g | fib 5g | carb 22g • serving size 1 packet of 3 mini cupcakes | ■

- Jell-O Sugar Free Mousse Temptations
  cal 60 | fat 3g | fib 0g | carb 9g • serving size 1 cup | ■

* • Jell-O Sugar Free Pudding Mix (made with nonfat milk)
  cal 97 | fat 0g | fib 0g | carb 6g • serving size 1/2 cup | ■

* • Jelly Belly Sugar Free Jelly Beans
  cal 80 | fat .5g | fib 1g | carb 37g • serving size 1/2 bag | ■

- Kashi 7 Whole Grain Puffs
  cal 88 | fat 1g | fib 3g | carb 15g • serving size 1 cup | ■

- Keebler Waffle Bowls or Waffle Cones
  cal 50 | fat 1g | fib 0g | carb 10g • serving size 1 bowl or cone | ■

- Kens or Wishbone Salad Spritzers
  cal 10/15 | fat 0g | fib 0g | carb 2g • serving size 10 sprays | □

* • Kix Cereal
  cal 88 | fat 1g | fib 3g | carb 15g • serving size 1 cup | ■

- Krusteaz Muffin Mix (asst'd varieties)
  cal 140 | fat 0g | fib 2g | carb 31g • serving size muffin | ■ ■

- Kudos M&M Granola Bars
  cal 100 | fat 3g | fib 1g | carb 17g • serving size 1 bar | ■ ■

- Little Debbie Pecan Spinwheels
  cal 100 | fat 1g | fib 0g | carb 16g • serving size 1 sweet roll | ■

- Moo Magic Milk Mix (assorted flavors)
  cal 5 | fat 0g | fib 0g | carb 1g • serving size 1 packet | □

- Motts Plus Fiber Apple Sauce (asst'd flavors)
  cal 50 | fat 0g | fib 3g | carb 15g • serving size 1 container | □

- Musselman's Lite Apple Sauce
  cal 50 | fat 0g | fib 2g | carb 12g • serving size 1 container | ■

- Nabisco 100 Calorie Snack Packs (assorted varieties)
  cal 100 | fat 3g | fib 0g | carb 17g • serving size 1 snack pack | ■ ■

- Nonnis Biscotti (assorted varieties)
  cal 110 | fat 4.5g | fib 1g | carb 17g • serving size 1 biscotti | ■ ■

- Ocean Spray, Diet Cranberry
  cal 5 | fat 0g | fib 0g | carb 3g • serving size 8 fl oz | □

- Ocean Spray, Diet Grape
  cal 5 | fat 0g | fib 0g | carb 2g • serving size 8 fl oz | □

- Old El Paso Refried Beans, fat free
  cal 100 | fat 0g | fib 6g | carb 18g • serving size 1/2 cup | □

- Old El Paso Refried Beans, spicy fat free
  cal 90 | fat 0g | fib 5g | carb 16g • serving size 1/2 cup | ■

- Olde Cape Cod Fat Free Salad Dressings (asst'd. varieties)
  cal 40 | fat 0g | fib 0g | carb 9g • serving size 2 tbsp | ■

- Ortega Whole Grain Corn Taco Shells
  cal 55 | fat 3g | fib 3 | carb 8g • serving size 1 taco shell | ■

* • Pickles, Dill or Sugar-Free Sweet
  cal 0 | fat 0g | fib 0g | carb 0g • serving size 1 oz | □

- Progresso Light Soups
  cal 60 | fat 0g | fib 4g | carb 22g • serving size 1 cup | □

* • Puffin Original Cereal
  cal 90 | fat 1g | fib 5g | carb 23g • serving size 3/4 cup | ■

- Ragu Light Fat Free Sauce Tomato & Basil
  cal 50 | fat 0g | fib 2g | carb 11g • serving size 1/2 cup | ■

- Ragu Light No Sugar Added Sauce Tomato & Basil
  cal 50 | fat 1g | fib 3g | carb 9g • serving size 1/2 cup | □

- Roasted Red Peppers–no oil
  cal 5 | fat 0g | fib 0g | carb 1g • serving size 1 oz | □

- Ronzoni Healthy Harvest Pasta
  cal 180 | fat 2g | fib 6g | carb 42g • serving size 2 oz dry | ■ ■ ■

- Salsa (many brands)
  cal 15 | fat 0g | fib 0g | carb 3g • serving size 2 tbsp | □

- Sipahh Milk Flavoring Straws (assorted varieties)
  cal 15 | fat 0g | fib 0g | carb 3g • serving size 1 straw | □

* • Smart Beat Mayonnaise
  cal 10 | fat 0g | fib 0g | carb 3g • serving size 1 tbsp | □

- Special K Bars (asst'd flavors)
  cal 90 | fat 2g | fib 0g | carb 17g • serving size 1 bar | ■ ■

* • Splenda Flavor Blends for Coffee
  cal 0 | fat 0g | fib 0g | carb 0g • serving size 1 packet | □

- StarKist Chunk Light Tuna in Water
  cal 90 | fat 1g | fib 1g | carb 1g • serving size 3 oz foil pouch | ■ ■

- St. Dalfour Gourmet on the Go Pasta & Vegetables
  cal 100 | fat 3g | fib 4g | carb 13g • serving size 1/2 can | ■

- Swanson White Chicken Breast in Water
  cal 70 | fat 1g | fib 0g | carb 2g • serving size 3 oz can | ■

- Sushi Chef Panko (Japanese Bread Flakes)
  cal 90 | fat .5g | fib 3g | carb 19g • serving size 1/2 cup | ■

- Thin Ribbon Candy
  cal 60 | fat 0g | fib 0g | carb 15g • serving size 1 long piece | ■

- Torani Flavored Syrups
  cal 0 | fat 0g | fib 0g | carb 0g • serving size 1 oz | □

- Vermont Sugar Free Maple Syrup
  cal 15 | fat 0g | fib 0g | carb 5g • serving size 1/4 cup | □

*• VitaBrownie Mix
  cal 90 | fat 1.5g | fib 7g | carb 21g • serving size 1 brownie | ■

- VitaMuffin Mix
  cal 100 | fat 1.5g | fib 6g | carb 19g • serving size 1 muffin | ■

- Wasa Crisp'n Light 7 Grain Cracker Bread
  cal 60 | fat 0g | fib 2g | carb 13g • serving size 3 crackers | ■

- Welch's Light Grape
  cal 50 | fat 0g | fib 0g | carb 13g • serving size 8 oz | ■

- Wishbone or Ken's Salad Spritzers
  cal 10/15 | fat 5g | fib 0g | carb 2g • serving size 10 sprays/1g | □

- V-8 Diet Splash
  cal 10 | fat 0g | fib 0g | carb 3g • serving size 8 oz | □

- V-8 V-Fusion Light
  cal 50 | fat 0g | fib 0g | carb 13g • serving size 8 oz | ■

- Walden Farms No Carbs Alfredo Sauce
  cal 0 | fat 0g | fib 0g | carb 0g • serving size 3 tbsp | □

MEATS/SEAFOOD

- Ball Park Smoked White Turkey Franks
  cal 45 | fat 0g | fib 0g | carb 5g • serving size 1 frank | ■

- Butterball Deli Thin Sliced Chicken Breast
  cal 50 | fat .5g | fib 0g | carb 1g • serving size 4 slices | ■

- Chesapeake Bay Low Fat Crab Cakes
  cal 80 | fat 1.5g | fib 0g | carb 9g • serving size 1 cake | ■ ■

* • Eckrich Ready Crisp Fully-Cooked Bacon
  cal 47 | fat 4g | fib 0g | carb 0g • serving size 2 slices | ■

- Gorton's Grilled Fish Fillets (assorted flavors)
  cal 100 | fat 3g | fib 0g | carb 1g • serving size 1 fillet | ■ ■

- Healthy Choice Polish Kielbasa
  cal 80 | fat 2.5g | fib 0g | carb 6g • serving size 2 oz | ■ ■

- Healthy Ones Turkey/Ham Slices
  cal 60 | fat 1.5g | fib 0g | carb 2g • serving size 7 slices | ■

- Hebrew National 97% Fat Free Beef Hot Dogs
  cal 40 | fat 1g | fib 0g | carb 3g • serving size 1 dog | ■

- Hormel Turkey Pepperoni
  cal 70 | fat 4g | fib 0g | carb 0g • serving size 17 slices | ■ ■

- Hormel Turkey Pepperoni Minis
  cal 70 | fat 4g | fib 0g | carb 0g • serving size 1 oz | ■ ■

- Ken's Cocktail Sauce
  cal 70 | fat 2g | fib 1g | carb 13g • serving size 1/4 cup | ■

- Natures Place Chicken Sausage
  cal 90 | fat 4.5g | fib 0g | carb 1g • serving size 1 link | ■ ■

* • Oscar Mayer Fully Cooked Bacon
  cal 52.5 | fat 4.5g | fib 0g | carb 0g • serving size 3 slices | ■

- Oscar Mayer 98% Fat Free Deli Meat (asst'd)
  cal 45 | fat .5g | fib 0g | carb 2g • serving size 6 slices | ■

* • Oscar Mayer 98% Fat Free Weiners
  cal 40 | fat 1g | fib 0g | carb 3g • serving size 1 dog | ■

- Purdue Short Cuts Honey Roasted Chicken Breast
  cal 90 | fat 2g | fib 0g | carb 2g • serving size 1/2 cup | ■ ■

- Sea Choice Salmon Burger
  cal 100 | fat 1.5g | fib 0g | carb 5g • serving size 1 burger | ■ ■

* • Shrimp, Fresh or Frozen (71/90 count)
  cal 60 | fat .5g | fib 0g | carb 2g • serving size 16 shrimp (3 oz) | ■

- Tyson Fajita Chicken Breast Strips
  cal 100 | fat 2g | fib 0g | carb 2g • serving size 3 oz | ■ ■

- Yakinori Hanedashi Toasted Seaweed Sheets
  cal 5 | fat 0g | fib 0g | carb 1g • serving size 1 sheet | ☐

DAIRY / REFRIGERATOR

(some may be located in deli section)

* *• 8th Continent Light Vanilla Soy Milk
  cal 60 | fat 2g | fib 0g | carb 5g • serving size 8 oz | ■

* • Alpine Lace Reduced Fat Provolone
  cal 60 | fat 4.5g | fib 0g | carb 1g • serving size 1 slice | ■ ■

* • Boursin Light Garlic & Herb Cheese
  cal 40 | fat 2.5g | fib 0g | carb 3g • serving size 1⅔ tbsp | ■

* • Brummel & Brown Buttery Spread
  cal 45 | fat 5g | fib 0g | carb 0g • serving size 1 tbsp | ■

* • Cabot 75% Light Cheddar Cheese
  cal 60 | fat 2.5g | fib 0g | carb <1g • serving size 1 oz | ■

* *• Calabro Fat Free Ricotta
  cal 60 | fat 0g | fib 0g | carb 1g • serving size 1/2 cup | ■

* • Coffee Mate Coffee Creamer, Fat Free
  cal 25 | fat 0g | fib 0g | carb 5g • serving size 1 tbsp | □

* • Coffee Mate Coffee Creamer, Sugar Free
  cal 15 | fat 1g | fib 0g | carb 1g • serving size 1 tbsp | □

* • Dannon Light & Fit Carb Control Yogurt
  cal 50 | fat 3g | fib 0g | carb 3g • serving size 4 oz cup | ■

* • Dannon Light & Fit Smoothie
  cal 70 | fat 0g | fib 0g | carb 13g • serving size 7 oz | ■

* • Dannon Light & Fit Yogurt
  cal 80 | fat 0g | fib 0g | carb 10g • serving size 6 oz | ■ ■

* • Egg Beaters
  cal 30 | fat 0g | fib 0g | carb 1g • serving size 1/4 cup | ■

* • Gatorade G-2
  cal 25 | fat 0g | fib 0g | carb 7g • serving size 8 oz | □

* *• Half & Half, Fat Free (most brands)
  cal 20 | fat 0g | fib 0g | carb 3g • serving size 2 tbsp | □

* • Hood Fat Free Cottage Cheese with Pineapple
  cal 100 | fat 0g | fib 0g | carb 15g • serving size 1/2 cup | ■ ■

We always have time for our priorities.

- *• I Can't Believe It's Not Butter
  cal 0 | fat 0g | fib 0g | carb 0g • serving size 5 sprays | □

- • Jarlsberg Lite Reduced Fat Swiss Cheese Deli Thin Sliced
  cal 50 | fat 2.5g | fib 0g | carb 0g • serving size 1 slice | ■

- • Jell-O Sugar Free Pudding Snacks
  cal 60 | fat 1g | fib 0g | carb 13g • serving size 1 snack cup | ■

- • Kozy Shack No Sugar Added Puddings
  (Tapioca & Chocolate)
  cal 90 | fat 3g | fib 4g | carb 11g • serving size 1 snack cup | ■

- • Kozy Shack No Sugar Added Black Forest Puddings
  cal 70 | fat 2g | fib 3g | carb 9g • serving size 1 snack cup | ■

- • Kraft Fat Free Shredded Cheddar or Mozzarella
  cal 45 | fat 0g | fib 0g | carb 2g • serving size 1/4 cup | ■

- *• Laughing Cow Cheese Wedges (assorted flavors)
  cal 35 | fat 2g | fib 0g | carb 1g • serving size 1 wedge | ■

- *• Laughing Cow Gourmet Cheese & Baguettes
  cal 60 | fat 3.5g | fib 1g | carb 5g • serving size 1 cheese & cracker unit | ■

- • Mini Baby Bell Light Semi Soft Cheese
  cal 50 | fat 3g | fib 0g | carb 0g • serving size 1 piece | ■

- *• Pillsbury Cinnamon Rolls With Icing, Reduced Fat
  cal 140 | fat 3.5g | fib 0g | carb 24g • serving size 1 roll | ■ ■ ■

- • Pillsbury Dinner Rolls, Low Fat
  cal 110 | fat 1.5g | fib 0g | carb 19g • serving size 1 roll | ■ ■

- *• President's Crumbled Fat Free Feta (assorted varieties)
  cal 60 | fat 0g | fib 0g | carb 4g • serving size 2 oz | ■

- *• Smart Balance or I Can't Believe It's Not Butter Spray
  cal 0 | fat 0g | fib 0g | carb 0g • serving size 5 sprays | □

- *• Sonoma Jacks Cheese Wedges, asst'd flavors
  cal 25–50 | fat 1.5–3g | fib 0g | carb 1g • serving size 1 wedge | ■

- • Sour Cream, Fat Free (many brands)
  cal 20–30 | fat 0g | fib 0g | carb 3g • serving size 2 tbsp | □

- • Trader Joe's Fat Free Crumbled Feta Cheese
  cal 35 | fat 0g | fib 0g | carb 2g • serving size 1 oz | ■

- • Tropicana Light & Healthy Orange Juice
  cal 50 | fat 0g | fib 0g | carb 13g • serving size 8 oz | ■

- Weight Watchers String Cheese
  cal 50 | fat 2.5g | fib 0g | carb 1g • serving size 1 | ■

- Weight Watchers Yogurt (assorted varieties)
  cal 100 | fat .5g | fib 3g | carb 17g • serving size 6 oz | ■

BREADS

(some may be located in deli section)

- Arnold's Sandwich Thins
  cal 100 | fat 1g | fib 5g | carb 22g • serving size 1 | ■

- Beefsteak Light Rye Bread
  cal 80 | fat 1g | fib 5g | carb 20g • serving size 2 slices | ■

* • Cedar's Lavash Bread
  cal 100 | fat 5g | fib 6g | carb 7g • serving size 1 (9 x 12) lavash | ■ ■

- Cedar's Whole Wheat Roll-Ups
  cal 90 | fat 4g | fib 5g | carb 14g • serving size 1 roll-up | ■

* • Flatout Light Flatbread (Original, Italian Herb, Sundried Tomato)
  cal 90 | fat 2.5g | fib 9g | carb 16g • serving size 1 flatbread | ■

- Joseph's Flax, Oat Bran & Whole Wheat Lavash Bread
  cal 100 | fat 4g | fib 6g | carb 14g • serving size 1 (9 x 12) lavash | ■ ■

- Joseph's Flax, Oat Bran & Whole Wheat Pitas
  cal 45 | fat 1g | fib 4g | carb 8g • serving size 1 (1-oz) pita | ■

- Joseph's Oat Bran & Whole Wheat Tortillas
  cal 70 | fat 1.5g | fib 6g | carb 11g • serving size 1 tortilla | ■

* • Kim's Flat Breads
  cal 100 | fat 4g | fib 6g | carb 14g • serving size 1/2 flat bread | ■

* • Kim's Light Bagels (assorted flavors)
  cal 110 | fat 1g | fib 4g | carb 22g • serving size 1 bagel | ■

- LaTortilla Factory Whole Wheat Tortillas
  cal 90 | fat 3g | fib 14g | carb 19g • serving size 1 tortilla | ■

- Light Breads (most brands)
  cal 80 | fat 0g | fib 6g | carb 20g • serving size 2 slices | ■

- Light English Muffins (most brands)
  cal 90 | fat 0g | fib 6g | carb 21g • serving size 1 muffin | ■

- Marzetti Fat Free Garlic & Onion Croutons
  cal 60 | fat 0g | fib 0g | carb 10g • serving size 4 tbsp | ■

- Melissa's Crepes
  cal 51 | fat 1g | fib 0g | carb 9g • serving size 1 crepe | ■

- Pepperidge Farms Deli Flats
  cal 100 | fat 1.5g | fib 5g | carb 20g • serving size 1 roll | ■

- Thomas' Light Multi-Grain English Muffins
  cal 100 | fat 1g | fib 8g | carb 24g • serving size 1 muffin | ■

- Tumaro's Low Carb Wraps (assorted varieties)
  cal 50 | fat 1.5g | fib 1g | carb 4g • serving size 1 wrap | ■

- Weight Watchers Whole Wheat Pita
  cal 100 | fat 1g | fib 9g | carb 24g • serving size 1 pita | ■

FROZEN FOODS

- Alexia Oven Reds potatoes
  cal 120 | fat 3.5g | fib 2g | carb 19g • serving size 3 oz | ■ ■

* • Athens Fillo Dough
  cal 36 | fat 0g | fib 0g | carb 8g • serving size 1 sheet | ■

- Athens Mini Fillo Shells
  cal 60 | fat 3g | fib 0g | carb 6g • serving size 3 shells | ■

- Birds Eye Steamfresh Asian Style Chicken Veg Medley
  cal 290 | fat 6g | fib 10g | carb 36g • serving size 1/2 bag | ■ ■ ■ ■ ■

- Breyers No Sugar Added Double Churned Vanilla
  cal 80 | fat 4g | fib 4g | carb 14g • serving size 1/2 cup | ■

* • Cool Whip, Fat Free
  cal 15 | fat 0g | fib 0g | carb 3g • serving size 2 tbsp | □

- Earth's Best Organic Mini Waffles
  cal 80 | fat 3g | fib 2g | carb 12g • serving size 4 mini waffles | ■

- Edy's Slow Churned—No Sugar Added (Vanilla, Coffee, Neopolitan)
  cal 90 | fat 3g | fib 2g | carb 13g • serving size 1/2 cup | ■ ■

- Eggo's Nutri-Grain Low Fat Waffles
  cal 70 | fat 1g | fib 1.5g | carb 13g • serving size 1 waffle | ■

* • Gardenburgers Veggie Medley
  cal 90 | fat 3g | fib 5g | carb 15g • serving size 1 burger | ■

- Green Giant Healthy Heart
  cal 140 | fat 3g | fib 4g | carb 28g • serving size 7 oz box | ■ ■

- Healthy Choice Premium Ice Cream Bars
  cal 80 | fat 1g | fib 4g | carb 13g • serving size 1 bar | ■

- Hood Sugar Free Light Whipped Cream
  cal 10 | fat .5g | fib 0g | carb <1g • serving size 2 tbsp | □

- Lean Pockets Sausage, Egg, Cheese
  cal 150 | fat 4.5g | fib 2g | carb 19g • serving size 1 breakfast pocket | ■■

- Luigi's Real Italian Ice (assorted varieties)
  cal 130 | fat 0g | fib 0g | carb 33g • serving size 1 ice | ■■

- McCain Roasters—Potatoes
  cal 120 | fat 3g | fib 2g | carb 22g • serving size 3 oz | ■■

- McCain Roasters—Sweet Potato Fries
  cal 120 | fat 3g | fib 2g | carb 22g • serving size 3 oz | ■■

- Ore-Ida Steam n Mash Potatoes
  cal 80 | fat 0g | fib 0g | carb 17g • serving size 3/4 cup | ■■

- Skinny Cow Giant Fudge Bars
  cal 100 | fat 1g | fib 4g | carb 22g • serving size 1 bar | ■

- Skinny Cow Ice Cream Sandwiches (assorted flavors)
  cal 140 | fat 1.5g | fib 3g | carb 30g • serving size 1 sandwich | ■■

- Tropicana Light Fruit & Cream Bars
  cal 45 | fat .5g | fib 4g | carb 14g • serving size 1 bar | □

*• Turkey Hill No Sugar Added Fat Free Vanilla Ice Cream
  cal 70 | fat 0g | fib 5g | carb 20g • serving size 1/2 cup | ■

- Tyson Breast Tenderloins
  cal 150 | fat 7g | fib 1g | carb 12g • serving size 1 tenderloin | ■■■

- Tyson Grilled Chicken Strips
  cal 100 | fat 1.5g | fib 0g | carb 3g • serving size 3 oz | ■■

- Van's 97% Fat Free Waffles
  cal 75 | fat 1g | fib 2.5g | carb 15g • serving size 1 waffle | ■

*• Vita Muffins & Tops (assorted varieties)
  cal 100 | fat 1.5g | fib 6g | carb 24g • serving size 1 muffin | ■

*• Weight Watchers Giant Fudge Bars
  cal 110 | fat 1g | fib 5g | carb 25g • serving size 1 bar | ■

acknowledgments

I want to thank . . .

Aleeta, Adam, Alan, and Andrew, *the best children a mom could have.* Thanks for your encouragement, love, and laughter. I praise God for you every day.

My precious dad, David Cobb, Sr. See me, Dad? I really am your little girl now!

My mom, Mary Voyer, and her fab new husband, Clement. Mom, I'll never understand how you knew I would one day do it! Thanks for believing.

My incredible sister, Heather Lutz, who is always there for me and has more godly wisdom than a bratty little sister should. Love you, sis! NNBILYM.

My brother, David Cobb, Jr., whom I've adored since I could walk. Thanks for all your help with bagels!

My grandparents, Bick and Marlene Stevens . . . the first WW Life-time Members in our family . . . you showed me it could be done. (Grampy died during the writing of *Finally Thin!* I love you, Grampy! Keep counting those points!)

My selfless, loving aunt, Tina Scharback, and the rest of my wonderfully supportive family:
Agnes Bensen (whose kind inheritance funded Kim's Light Bagels. Thanks, Bestemore!), Jean Bensen, Alan and Lisa Bensen, and all the

other Bensens, Huffs, Lutzs, Olsens, Scharbacks, Streits, and Teasdales. You're all crazy and I love you!

My best friend, Cathy Getz. Thanks for walking this journey with me. It was fun, wasn't it?

And my dear friend Peter Pough. Who knew when you became my WW receptionist years ago that you would be Kim Bensen Enterprises' first employee! I would have quit long ago without you! Let's always keep it fun. :-) Thanks, P . . . catch!

Penny Pompa, whose talents in the kitchen are far superior to mine. You keep me sane. P.S. I love it when you snort when you laugh.

Karen Tuzzio, thanks for figuring out my books and putting up with the endless piles of receipts.

Matt Bazan, you created so much out of so little. Thanks for pushing. I'm better for it.

Jenn Gallo-McPhatter—Wow! Thank you for giving me daylight back.

Pastor Dave and Andrea McIntyre, Gail Sullivan, and the rest of my Calvary Church family—I am so grateful. Phil 1: 3–6.

My literary agent, Coleen O'Shea, for meeting me for coffee, listening to my story, and taking a chance on this very inexperienced first-time author. You're great!

Everyone on my Random House team.

Barbara Alpert, a wonderful editor and cohort in dieting. You made *Finally Thin!* so much better. Thanks.

To all my wonderful Kimmies, monkees, Wednesday night buddies, back row and really cuuuuute members whom I love so much. You keep me grounded and give back to me so much more than I could ever give to you. You can do it!

Dianne Doctor: I won't forget. Lou Doctor: Many happy returns.

Most of all I thank my Lord and Savior Jesus Christ.

In my anguish I cried to the Lord and
He answered by setting me free.

—Psalm 118:5

about the author

Kim Bensen lives in Shelton, Connecticut,
with her husband and four children.

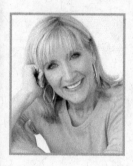

If you feel ready to begin *your* weight loss
journey and would like some support, head
to www.kimbensen.com/store/membership.
Enter the promo code FINALLYTHIN at
check out and get started with a free four-
week complimentary membership. *I know
you can do it. I'd love to help.*